# HOW TO LIVE WELL WITH EARLY ALZHEIMER'S

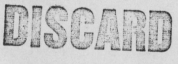

## Books in the Healthy Home Library Series
## from St. Martin's Paperbacks

# HOW TO LIVE WELL
# WITH EARLY
# ALZHEIMER'S

## Deborah Mitchell

A Lynn Sonberg Book

St. Martin's Paperbacks

Notice: This book is intended as a reference volume only, not as a medical manual. The information given here is designed to help you make informed decisions about your health. It is not intended as a substitute for any treatment that may have been prescribed by your doctor. If you suspect that you have a medical problem, we urge you to seek competent medical help.

Mention of specific companies, organizations, or authorities in this book does not imply endorsement by the author or publisher, nor does mention of specific companies, organizations, or authorities imply that they endorse this book, its author or the publisher.

Internet addresses given in this book were accurate at the time it went to press.

HOW TO LIVE WELL WITH EARLY ALZHEIMER'S

Copyright © 2010 by Lynn Sonberg Book Associates.

All rights reserved.

For information address St. Martin's Press, 175 Fifth Avenue, New York, NY 10010.

EAN: 978-0-312-37316-0

Printed in the United States of America

St. Martin's Paperbacks edition / March 2010

St. Martin's Paperbacks are published by St. Martin's Press, 175 Fifth Avenue, New York, NY 10010.

10  9  8  7  6  5  4  3  2  1

# CONTENTS

# HOW TO LIVE WELL
# WITH EARLY
# ALZHEIMER'S

# INTRODUCTION

This is a book about action, hope, love, and perseverance. It is also about a disease that strikes fear into the hearts and minds of millions of people, a fear so strong for some that they will not even utter the words "Alzheimer's disease," nor seek help when they suspect it has affected them or someone they love.

Yet we cannot be silent about this condition. Every 70 seconds, someone develops Alzheimer's disease. Currently, Alzheimer's affects approximately 5.3 million people in the United States, and experts project that by 2050, the number may rise to 30 million in the United States and 100 million around the world.

And there is one more thing we cannot be silent about: It is important to identify this disease in its earliest stages, because you *can* live well with early Alzheimer's disease.

One reason we can say these things is that there is a constant flow of research being conducted and reported on Alzheimer's disease. It is not unusual to hear news reports several times a week about cutting-edge diagnostic techniques, studies of medications and natural remedies, reports on therapy techniques, and investigations into what causes the disease. Thus far this flurry of activity has not generated a cure for the disease, but many scientists and researchers believe it is just a matter of time. And until then, they are finding and reporting on ways to make living with Alzheimer's disease as comfortable and positive as possible, as well as ways to prevent development of the disease.

That's where this book comes in. We take a look at the latest information about memory, memory loss, and Alzheimer's disease. We explore and explain the tried-and-true, up-and-coming, and sometimes experimental ways you or your loved ones can live well with early Alzheimer's disease. We discuss changes you can make to your lifestyle and actions you can take to help ward off or prevent memory loss and dementia, things that can also improve your quality of life.

For example, the use of brain exercises is so important, we have dedicated an entire chapter to it. These easy, often entertaining activities are effective not only in slowing progression of memory loss in people who have Alzheimer's, but also in preventing memory loss in people who do not have the disease. We also discuss various complementary medicine practices that can not only enhance the value of medications typically prescribed for Alzheimer's disease, but also improve quality of life for both the patient and his or her caregiver. We also dedicate a chapter to activities designed to improve the daily lives of people who have early Alzheimer's disease, including music, gardening, dance, and yoga.

All of these things, and more, can help you or your loved one live well, and perhaps longer, with early Alzheimer's disease. The phrase "early Alzheimer's disease" does not have a definitive length of time assigned to it. Although some experts say early Alzheimer's usually lasts only a couple of years, others, like Gayatri Devi, M.D., author of *What Your Doctor May* Not *Tell You about*

*Alzheimer's Disease* and director of the New York Memory and Healthy Aging Services, has treated patients with Alzheimer's who have maintained good function for five or six years or longer. The point is, although the length of time of early Alzheimer's may be uncertain, providing stimulating, enjoyable, and preventive activities and remedies along the way will most certainly improve qualify of life during whatever time there is.

All these things can be done, if you give them a chance.

And who are you? Because you picked up this book, you may be someone who has early Alzheimer's disease, someone who is experiencing some memory loss and wants to do something about it, someone who has a family member or other loved one who has early Alzheimer's disease, or an individual who cares for someone who has the disease. This book is for all of you, and it is our hope that it can help you take positive steps to improve the quality of life of someone who has early Alzheimer's disease and those who love him or her.

# PART I
The Art and Science of Diagnosis

# CHAPTER 1

What Is Memory?

Oscar Wilde once said, "Memory is the diary we all carry about with us," and this sentiment presents a familiar, convenient image. But you can't hold a memory, like you can a diary. Nor can you taste it, smell it, see it, or hear it. A touch can, however, be the stimulus that causes a memory to come to your consciousness. The same is true of a smell, a sound, a scene, or a food or beverage. But none of these concepts answers the big questions: *What is memory? How does the human brain collect, store, and process memories? Where does memory go when it's "gone"?*

Chances are one of the reasons you are holding this book is that these are some of the very questions you are asking yourself, perhaps for yourself or for a loved one who is experiencing memory loss or who has early Alzheimer's disease. It's also very likely that you also want to know what you can do about preventing and preserving memory. But before we can answer any of these and other related questions and concerns, it's helpful to have a basic understanding of how a healthy brain works.

# HOW A HEALTHY BRAIN WORKS

The human brain is a three-pound biological wonder. The estimated 100 billion nerve cells (neurons) that populate this soft, grayish-white mass dictate nearly everything you do whether you are conscious of it or not. Thus your brain controls not only the love you feel for your partner but the beating of your heart whenever you see him or her.

The vast amount of research into the causes, prevention, and treatment of Alzheimer's disease and other dementias goes hand-in-hand with the work being done by scientists to explore the extremely complex workings of the brain. Here is some of what we know thus far about the brain and how it works.

The brain loves sugar (glucose), and it needs a constant supply of this food to nourish and energize the constant activity of the billions of neurons. Let's liken this activity to a relay race. The neurons have fibers (called dendrites and axons) that form connections with other nerve cells. When a nerve cell is activated (as when we hear the starting gun at the start of a race), it sends an electrical message (like a baton) along the length of a long fiber called an axon.

When the signal reaches the end of the nerve cell (the handing-off point), brain chemicals called neurotransmitters are released from another type of fiber called dendrites. The neurotransmitters cross the gap between nerve cells (synapses) and attach themselves to receptors on the nerve cell on the other side of the synapse. Nerve cells that accept neurotransmitters (accept the baton from the "runner") then pass the message along to the next nerve cell, and on and on until the signal reaches its end point.

When you keep repeating an action (for example, practicing a tennis serve), you restimulate and reactivate the same nerve cell connections, or synapses, again and again. After you have practiced for some time, the synapses undergo a physical change and become stronger and more efficient at storing the behavior in your long-term memory. The areas of the brain that form the core of the memory-processing center are the hippocampus, the amygdala, and several other structures in the temporal lobe.

The hippocampus lies deep within the brain in the temporal lobe. Experts generally agree that the hippocampus plays a critical role in the formation of new memories of events (episodic memory). It is one of the first areas of the brain to suffer damage in people who have Alzheimer's disease.

The amygdala appears to have an important part in the formation of emotional memory. As you will learn below, emotional memory is very powerful and long-lasting.

## WHAT IS MEMORY?

Memory is a brain function that involves the ability to retain information or to recover information about experiences from the past. When we say or think to ourselves, "I remember that!" there is a process that takes place in the brain that involves the recovery and reconstruction of information that we have stored about things we have learned or done.

### Types of Memory

Memory can be broken down into three categories: sensory, short-term, and long-term. **Sensory memory** occurs when you first encounter or perceive an event or object. For example, let's say you are driving in an unfamiliar city and you get lost. The moment you realize you do not know where you are, you are overtaken by a feeling of anxiety and frustration. A sensory memory has just been created.

**Short-term memory** (also known as working memory) stores information that you need to remember within a short amount of time (minutes to hours). Now that you are lost, you decide you need to stop to ask someone for directions. When you receive the verbal direction, you will need to retrieve the instructions while you maneuver through the streets. This information is short-term memory.

Chances are you won't need to remember the directions again and again, so your memory of them will eventually be replaced by other memories. That is the nature of short-term memories: They are supposed to be fleeting. If they were not, you would not be able to accommodate them. Research shows that the average person is able to retain only about seven (plus or minus two) unrelated pieces of information in the mind at one time. That's why it's easier to remember a seven-digit telephone number or a Social Security number rather than a vehicle identification number or a set of complicated directions on how to break down and reassemble a motor.

Short-term memory also is fragile. Let's return to the driving example. If while you are getting verbal directions your passenger interrupts you by saying, "Do you think we'll make it by two-thirty, because I have an appointment," chances are you will forget some or all of the instructions being given to you. This mental glitch is normal; it is simply the nature of short-term memory. We will be referring to short-term memory often, as this is a type of memory that is lost by people who have Alzheimer's disease. For example, it is typical for individuals in the early stages of Alzheimer's to forget what they had for lunch today, or to forget someone's name shortly after being told what it is.

In **long-term memory,** your brain stores information that you need to access again and again. In our example, long-term memory is your memory of how to drive. All long-term memory involves permanent, physical changes to the nerve cells and electrical circuitry of the brain. If you have ever wondered why a person who has moderate to severe Alzheimer's has poor or no short-term memory but can remember with clarity events from their childhood or the name of their first love, it is because their long-term memory is intact, "hardwired" into the brain.

Long-term memory can be broken down into three types, or parts:

- **Episodic memory** refers to the ability to recall personal events and experiences from the past. The past can be as recent as yesterday (remembering what you ate for lunch) or a baseball game you saw when you were seven years old. This type of memory organizes information around events (episodes) that occurred in your life. Episodic memory allows us to recall not only events but also information that is associated with those events. So, you may remember the baseball game as well as eating hot dogs and popcorn at the game. People who have early Alzheimer's disease generally have no problems with episodic memory.

- **Semantic** (or **declarative**) **memory** includes facts that are so entrenched in your brain that you don't have to exert any effort to recall them. Examples include knowing the days of the week or knowing what a cat is. This type of memory also allows people to understand written words regardless of what type style they are presented in, because the brain understands the concept of a letter rather than a specific example of one. These types of memories are subject to destruction early in Alzheimer's disease.

- **Procedural memory** is the type necessary to perform activities like driving, eating, dancing, and walking. It is the "how" type of long-term memory: the ability to remember how to do something in a series of steps. For driving, for example, those steps can include getting into the car, putting the key into the ignition, turning the key, putting the car into drive, and so on. When we retrieve information from procedural memory, we retrieve one step at a time, and each step then triggers the next step. Procedural memories are more resilient to destruction than are semantic memories in people who have Alzheimer's disease. Therefore, people in the early stages of the disease typically have little or no trouble remembering how to do the ballroom dancing they did for years, or how to make their favorite sandwich. Many people with early Alzheimer's disease even remember how to drive, although their sense of direction and remembering where they are going can be compromised and thus driving is often not safe for them to continue.

You may see different terms for these types of long-term memories, but overall, the consensus is that these various types of long-term memory are related and overlap, although scientists are not exactly sure how they work together.

The differences between short- and long-term memories are not simply how long the memories last. As we mentioned, the brain can only handle a small number of short-term memories at the same time, yet it can store an unlimited number of long-term memories. And unlike short-term memories, which are easily disrupted, long-term memories are not lost if some interrupt your train of thought.

## Memories and Emotions

Have you ever wondered why some memories stay clear for years while others fade over time? The answer is emotion, both positive and negative. Research shows that the brain retains many details about events that evoke lots of emotions (e.g., your wedding day, a traumatic car accident). In fact, according to a study done by experts at Duke University, women are more likely than men to report intense emotional experiences and to remember them.

Why does this happen? Two areas of the brain are active during successful retrieval of memories: the amygdala and the hippocampus. These areas of the brain are close to each other and they also successfully encode emotional memories. Therefore memories that have emotional significance for people are better hardwired in the brain and better recalled. So when your Aunt Helen can't remember what she had for lunch today but she can vividly remember the blue dress she wore the day she got her first kiss, you'll know why.

## What Do Memories Look Like?

A new study published in June 2009 by investigators at the Montreal Neurological Institute and Hospital, McGill University, and the University of California, Los Angeles states that for the first time, scientists have been able to capture an image that shows what happens when long-term memories are formed. What does long-term memory look like?

The researchers exposed nerve cells to a brain chemical called serotonin, which has been shown to stimulate the formation of memory. They then used a fluorescent protein capable of changing from green to red when it is exposed to ultraviolet light. When they flashed the cells with the light, they noted that any proteins that already existed turned red. But when they stimulated the cells to form

memories, they saw new green proteins under the micro-
scope.

Although green fluorescent blips may not be the stuff
of which poetry is written, this discovery is considered
a breakthrough for memory researchers. Images of long-
term memory are formed when new proteins are created at
the synapse, which is the connection between nerve cells.
When this action takes place, it increases the strength of the
synaptic connection and reinforces the memory that has
been formed. Neuroscientists now know that protein syn-
thesis is necessary for long-term memory to last. This information may help them develop new ways to prevent and
treat memory loss.

## Normal Memory Loss

Although it is common to think that memory problems
don't begin until people are middle-aged or older, the truth
is that brain cells begin to die when individuals are in
their twenties. This is also the time when the body makes
less of the chemicals the brain cells need to continue their
work. Over time, these brain cell changes begin to have
an impact on memory. Short-term and remote memories
are not usually impacted by the aging process, but recent
memory may be affected. Don't become alarmed if you
forget the names of people you were introduced to recently: This is part of normal changes in memory. In fact,
the more you fret over your inability to recall the names
immediately, the more difficult it may be for you to remember. That temporary lapse, however, is the result of
stress and not the onset of dementia. In most cases, you
will remember the names with time—perhaps minutes,
hours, or even a day or two.

When it comes to memory and memory loss, it is not a
matter of black and white, but plenty of gray areas in between. Caregivers of people who have Alzheimer's dis-

ease will often ask why their loved ones can remember something one day and then forget it the next, and then retrieve it again later. The answer, it seems, lies somewhere in that gray area.

Sometimes, however, memory problems persist and gradually grow worse, significantly affecting daily activities. You or a loved one may have trouble remembering how to do things that once were a habit or getting to a place that you have been to many times in the past. That's when you should stop and evaluate what is going on and ask, Is it Alzheimer's disease or is it something else? That's the question we address in the next chapter.

# CHAPTER 2

The Many Faces of Memory Loss

When people begin to notice lapses in their memory, too many believe that a diagnosis of Alzheimer's disease will inevitably follow. The truth, however, is that in many cases memory loss is caused by a reversible condition, or it may be attributed to a common condition known as mild cognitive impairment. In other people it is caused by a type of dementia besides Alzheimer's. The point is, if you have trouble remembering your shopping list, if you keep losing your keys, or if you can't remember someone's name, it doesn't necessarily mean the seeds of Alzheimer's disease or dementia have planted themselves in your brain.

In this chapter we explore the main causes of memory loss, namely aging, mild cognitive impairment (MCI), Alzheimer's disease, and other types of dementia, as well as use of medications, depression, alcoholism, medical conditions, and head trauma.

## AGE-RELATED MEMORY LAPSE

If you are age 50 or older, you are a member of a population in which about two-thirds of men and women notice memory problems, such as forgetting appointments, having trouble remembering names, and walking into a room and forgetting what they came for. Relax, these are small memory lapses that typically occur with age. These lapses—sometimes referred to as "senior moments"—may be frustrating, but they don't interfere with your ability to do your job, travel, run your household, or perform any of your other activities.

Several factors cause the brain to change in its ability to retrieve and hold onto memories. Along with the loss of neurons with age, older people often experience a decrease in blood flow to the brain. Less oxygen to the brain cells can mean a reduced ability to recall. The hippocampus is also very susceptible to age-related deterioration, and this can affect the ability to retain information.

Overall, age-related forgetfulness is not a loss of memory but a slowing down in the ability to absorb, store, and retrieve information. Thus, it might take you a little longer to recall someone's name or where a certain restaurant is located, but you will. Just be a little patient with yourself. If you begin to worry a lot about your senior moments, the stress itself can affect both memory functioning and mood. That's because the body releases cortisol, a hormone released by the adrenal glands in response to stress. High cortisol levels have a negative impact on memory, even in healthy individuals, and they can even damage the hippocampus.

Many brain functions, however, are barely affected by normal aging. For example, natural aging of the brain does not damage the knowledge and wisdom you've accumulated during your life, as well as your common sense, the ability to form reasonable arguments and judgments, and the ability to learn new skills (although it may take you a little longer to learn them).

At this point in their lives, some people who are experiencing age-related memory glitches take steps to exercise their brains as a precautionary measure against dementia and/or further cognitive deterioration. This is a positive move, and we strongly encourage it. In fact, the activities discussed in chapter 9 may provide you with some suggestions.

Contrary to what was once popular opinion, although brain cells begin to die when people are in their twenties, a healthy brain also keeps growing new neurons and creating new connections between them throughout people's lifespan. Studies show that people who continue to challenge themselves mentally and who keep learning increase their chances of retaining healthy brain function. Yes, you can teach an "old dog" new tricks!

## MILD COGNITIVE IMPAIRMENT

Mild cognitive impairment (MCI) is a condition in which a person experiences problems with memory, language, or other mental functions that are severe enough that other people notice them. These problems are also apparent on tests, but they are not serious enough to hinder daily activities or to meet the criteria for dementia.

If this definition seems a bit imprecise, you're right, but this is common when one is trying to diagnose a person's mental capacities. People who have been diagnosed with mild cognitive impairment basically have no problems with regular daily activities, such as dressing, shopping, and household chores, and they still maintain good reasoning and thinking skills. The most telling symptom of mild cognitive impairment is a decline in short-term memory that is worse than what is usually seen in people who have age-related memory problems.

## Rebecca's Story

Rebecca, for example, is a 65-year-old retired office manager whose husband, Peter, had noticed that she was having increasing problems remembering appointments and shopping items, and that she was writing notes to herself and leaving them around the house to remind herself of things she needed to do. She was also very easily distracted, and each time it happened she would forget what she was saying. This frustrated her, and the more she worried about her memory problems, the worse they seemed to get. Peter insisted his wife see a doctor, and they both entered the office hoping they would not hear the words "Alzheimer's disease."

After the doctor asked both Rebecca and Peter many questions about her symptoms and feelings, and then conducted a series of screening and diagnostic tests (which we discuss in chapter 3), she told the worried couple that Rebecca had mild cognitive impairment. Five years later, Rebecca and Peter are extremely pleased that neither has noticed any significant change in her memory, and they both continue to enjoy a fairly active lifestyle that includes travel and volunteering at a local homeless shelter.

## Mild Cognitive Impairment and Alzheimer's Disease

According to the American College of Physicians, MCI affects about 20 percent of people who are older than 70. Rebecca's doctor explained that people who have MCI are three times more likely to develop Alzheimer's or other dementias than people who do not have the impairment. Overall, about 50 percent of people who have MCI develop Alzheimer's disease within five years of their MCI diagnosis.

The good news is that about half of individuals who have MCI do *not* go on to develop Alzheimer's disease. Some people with MCI remain stable, and others even return to normal.

Currently there are no treatments for MCI that have been approved by the Food and Drug Administration (FDA), although studies are being conducted. We discuss some potential treatment approaches for MCI in chapter 4.

## Other Causes of Memory Loss

Several other conditions are associated with memory loss. Some are reversible; others are not. Here's a brief review of some reasons people experience memory loss that are not associated with aging, MCI, or dementias.

- **Depression**. Among otherwise healthy older adults, depression is a common complaint. Symptoms typically associated with depression include problems with memory, concentration, and clear thinking. Unfortunately, depression can sometimes be mistaken for early Alzheimer's disease or dementia, and one major reason for this mistake is that depression is often overlooked in the elderly and thus it is not treated. Therefore, anyone who appears to be depressed and who is also having memory difficulties should be evaluated for depression. Proper treatment can resolve memory issues.

- **Vitamin $B_{12}$ deficiency**. People age 60 and older are at increased risk of vitamin $B_{12}$ deficiency, and abnormally low levels of this nutrient can cause significant problems with memory, depression, mental confusion, irritability, and hallucinations. Older people are especially susceptible to vitamin $B_{12}$ deficiency because with age, the body loses some of its ability to properly absorb and utilize this vitamin. Supplementation, including injections of $B_{12}$ if necessary, can reverse memory problems.

- **Medical conditions**. Many different medical conditions have memory loss as one of its symptoms. Some of them include Parkinson's disease, stroke, head trauma, seizures, uremia, liver failure, herpes, meningitis, lupus, multiple sclerosis, brain tumors, and sepsis.

- **Hormone deficiencies**. Some studies show that women who have low estrogen levels may experience impaired thought processes and an increased risk of developing Alzheimer's disease. Based on the results of the Women's Health Initiative, which showed that use of hormone replacement therapy in postmenopausal women is associated with an increased risk of stroke, blood clots, and heart disease, most health-care practitioners do not believe that estrogen should be taken solely to protect against Alzheimer's disease. However, it is important to recognize that low estrogen levels may be why some older women experience memory problems. Research shows that estrogen may improve verbal memory in younger naturally postmenopausal women, and it also shows a negative effect of conjugated equine estrogen plus medrooxyprogesterone (e.g., Premarin) on verbal memory in younger and older postmenopausal women. Some experts recommend taking bioidentical estrogen (estrogen that is chemically identical to that produced by the body) rather than synthetic estrogen (which is typically prescribed and is found in Premarin and other drugs) to address memory issues.

- **Alcoholism**: According to the National Institute of Alcohol Abuse and Alcoholism, more than 17 million Americans are alcoholics or abuse alcohol. While moderate consumption of alcohol can enhance cognitive function and reduce the risk for memory loss and dementia, excessive drinking has an opposite effect. Research in rats has shown that low doses of alcohol can increase the release of a chemical called acetylcholine, which may improve memory. However, high doses of alcohol can inhibit the release of acetylcholine, and this may interfere with memory.

• **Drug/medication use**: Chronic use of certain over-the-counter and prescription drugs can have a negative impact on memory. As people age, bodily changes make it more likely that problems such as memory loss will result from medication use. Some of those changes include a reduced ability of the kidneys to remove drugs from the bloodstream as quickly as they can in younger people, slower metabolism of drugs by the liver (which increases their time in the body and thus influences their effects), and a greater ratio of fat to muscle, which increases the amount of time it takes to eliminate some drugs from the body. These factors need to be considered along with this fact: Older adults take an average of more than five prescription and three over-the-counter drugs at the same time. In geriatric clinics, the most common cause of reversible memory loss is a negative response to medications. Some medications that can cause memory loss are shown in the accompanying table. Anyone who is experiencing memory loss and who is also taking medications should bring all of their drugs to their physician and review them as a possible cause of the memory difficulties. Also bring along any nutritional or herbal supplements you are taking. While they may not cause memory loss, some can interact with medications, and your doctor should be aware of all the substances you are taking.

---

### Drugs That Can Cause Memory Loss

**Note:** This is only a representative list. Many drugs used to treat heart disease, hypertension, insomnia, depression, anxiety, seizures, and diabetes are associated with some degree of memory loss. Talk to your doctor about any medications you are taking and the risk of memory problems.

alprazolam (Xanax; up to 33% of people experience memory loss)

aripiprazole (Abilify)

atorvastatin (Lipitor)

benztropine mesylate (Cogentin)

bupropion hydrochloride (Wellbutrin, Zyban)

carbidopa, levodopa, and entacapone (Stalevo)

cimetidine (Tagamet)

clonazepam (Klonopin)

diazepam (Valium)

imatinib mesylate (Gleevec)

lamotrigine (Lamictal)

lisinopril (Prinivil)

lithium carbonate (Eskalith)

losartan (Cozaar)

losartan and hydrochlorothiazide (Hyzaar)

prednisone (Deltasone)

pregabalin (Lyrica)

ribavirin (Copaxone, Copegus)

rifampin and isoniazid (Rifamate)

scopolamine (Transderm Scop)

selegiline hydrochloride (Eldepryl)

sumatriptan succinate (Imitrex)

timolol and hydrochlorothiazide (Timolide)

topiramate (Topamax)

trazolam (Halcion)

tretinoin (Vesanoid)

zolpidem tartrate (Ambien)

zonisamide (Zonegran)

# ALZHEIMER'S DISEASE

Walter is a 70-year-old retired electrical engineer who is also an Impressionist art enthusiast. Since his retirement five years ago, Walter has spent much of his free time studying art and going to art galleries. He decided to incorporate his love of art into works of fiction, and he has already completed about a dozen short stories and is working on a historical art novel. Over the last year or so, he has noticed that it is increasingly difficult for him to organize his notes and to do the research necessary for his book. He tells his wife, Clara, that he feels like his brain is slowing down and that he can't remember names and dates all the time.

Six months ago, Walter and Clara had planned a three-week cruise, but as the time for the vacation approaches, Walter says he has changed his mind and doesn't want to go. He has become more and more depressed, and Clara has not yet convinced him to go to a doctor. Yet they both realize he should go, because Walter is displaying several of the early warning symptoms of Alzheimer's disease, a neurodegenerative disease (one in which neurons are destroyed) that mainly affects people who are 65 or older.

## What Is Alzheimer's Disease?

Alzheimer's disease is the most common type of **dementia**, which is a general term for a condition in which people lose memory and other mental abilities (e.g., concentration, reasoning, judgment, math skills) to such a degree that the losses interfere with daily functioning. The main characteristic of Alzheimer's disease is the progressive death of brain cells, a process that usually begins in the hippocampus. As you may recall, the hippocampus plays a critical role in the retrieval and storage of memories.

Scientists use imaging techniques such as magnetic resonance imaging (MRI) and positron emission tomography

(PET) to see the progression of cell death and Alzheimer's in the brain. (We discuss these and other imaging techniques in chapter 3.) The cell damage then usually expands to include the cerebral cortex, which includes the frontal, parietal, and temporal lobes. These are areas of the brain that process emotions, decision-making, and instincts and the ability to communicate and to perform simple tasks.

As the disease progresses overtime, the brain shrinks as an increasing number of brain cells die and synapses are destroyed. This process proceeds at a different rate for every person. The average course of the disease is eight to 10 years, but it can last for twice that long.

## Early- versus Late-onset Alzheimer's Disease

When Walter finally agreed to see a doctor, he was diagnosed with late-onset Alzheimer's disease, a form of the disease that affects between 90 and 95 percent of those who develop this type of dementia. People younger than 65—in fact, as young as 17—can be diagnosed with early-onset Alzheimer's, which affects between 5 and 10 percent of those who get the disease. Unlike late-onset Alzheimer's, the early form often runs in families, and many people with early-onset Alzheimer's have a parent or grandparent who also developed the disease at a young age. Another feature of early-onset Alzheimer's is that a significant proportion of the cases are linked to genetic mutations of three different chromosomes, numbers 1, 14, and 21.

## Tangles and Plaques

Two terms that are used a lot when talking about Alzheimer's disease are tangles and plaques. These words refer to the changes that take place in the brains of people who have Alzheimer's disease and are among the abnormal structures observed by Dr. Alois Alzheimer, the doctor who discovered this form of dementia.

Tangles are twisted fibers of a protein called tau. Healthy tau performs important tasks, such as transporting materials within nerve cells and helping the cells keep their shape. In Alzheimer's disease, however, tau twists into clumps and causes nerve cells to die.

Plaques are composed of a protein called beta-amyloid, which in a healthy state is excreted from the body. In people who have Alzheimer's, however, the beta-amyloid accumulates outside the nerve cells, damaging them and causing them to die. Beta-amyloid can also damage mitochondria, cell structures that produce energy for the cells. Damaged mitochondria produce other harmful substances called free radicals, which in turn cause oxidative stress. Recent research indicates that oxidative stress has a major part in Alzheimer's disease.

Yet another problem with the accumulation of beta-amyloid plaque is that it may cause an excessive amount of calcium to enter neurons and cause brain cells to die. This abnormal activity is not related to how much calcium you eat or take as supplements, so do not reduce your intake of calcium!

Both tangles and plaques tend to form in a predictable pattern, starting in areas of the brain that process memory and learning and then moving on to other regions. This movement follows the progression of Alzheimer's disease.

What causes healthy proteins like tau and beta-amyloid to turn "bad" and damage brain cells? This is one of the yet-unanswered questions about Alzheimer's disease and the topic of much research.

## Neurotransmitters and Alzheimer's Disease

A few other elements that are important in understanding Alzheimer's disease are neurotransmitters, chemicals that act as messengers in the brain. We need to mention them here, because we will be talking about them again when we discuss ways to treat Alzheimer's disease. Those neurotransmitters are:

- Acetylcholine: involved in creating and retrieving memories, as well as in attention and learning

- Dopamine: has a key role in mood, psychosis, and physical movement

- Glutamate: involved in long-term memory and learning

- Norepinephrine: has impact on emotions

- Serotonin: key player in depression, mood, and anxiety

## Signs and Symptoms of Alzheimer's Disease

One of the most important things to remember about Alzheimer's disease is that it typically progresses very slowly. Thus the signs and symptoms we talk about in this section may very likely come on insidiously. This fact, along with taking steps to help slow progression of the disease even further by following some of the suggestions we talk about in part 2, can significantly help individuals maintain their independence as long as possible.

According to the Alzheimer's Association, there are 10 signs and symptoms of the disease of which people should be aware. If you or anyone you know is experiencing any of these signs, please see a knowledgeable healthcare practitioner so you can get an accurate evaluation.

- Memory changes that disrupt daily life (e.g., forgetting important events and dates, asking the same questions again and again, always relying on notes to remember things)

• Challenges in planning and solving problems (e.g., difficulty with monthly bills and/or using a checkbook, trouble following a plan, like a recipe)

• Difficulty completing once familiar tasks (e.g., driving or the rules of a favorite game)

• Confusion with time or place (e.g., losing track of days and time, forgetting where you are or how you got there)

• Trouble understanding visual images and spatial relationships (e.g., judging distances, determining colors)

• New problems speaking or writing (e.g., trouble finding the right word, calling items by the wrong name)

• Misplacing items and losing the ability to retrace steps (e.g., putting shoes in the refrigerator)

• Withdrawal from work or social activities (e.g., removing yourself from social occasions, hobbies, etc.)

• Changes in mood and personality (e.g., becoming confused, fearful, depressed)

The changes in the brain that cause the signs and symptoms mentioned above begin years before the signs are evident to the affected individual and/or others. Ever-evolving new technologies are finding ways to detect these changes in the brain long before they are obvious. We talk about some of those technologies in chapter 3.

## Causes and Risk Factors

Experts know that Alzheimer's disease involves progressive death of brain cells, but they have not yet determined any one reason why these cells die. They have, however, identified certain risk factors that increase a person's chances of developing Alzheimer's. First let's look at risk factors you cannot change.

- **Age** is the greatest known risk factor for Alzheimer's. The likelihood of developing the disease increases with age: Most people who get the disease are 65 or older, and the likelihood doubles about every five years after age 65. The risk for people older than 85 is about 50 percent.

- **Family history** is a factor, increasing your risk if more than one family member has the disease. Research shows that people who have a parent, brother, sister, or child with Alzheimer's are more likely to get the disease themselves.

- **Genes** (genetics) can have a role in determining whether a person develops Alzheimer's. There are two types of genes in this regard: risk genes and deterministic genes. Risk genes increase the chances of developing the disease, but they do not mean a person is guaranteed to get it. So far scientists have identified one risk gene for Alzheimer's disease. Called apolipoprotein E-4 (APOE-4), it is one of three types of the APOE gene (APOE-2 and APOE-3 are the other two). People who inherit one copy of the APOE-4 gene have an increased risk of developing the disease. If you have inherited two copies, your risk increases more, but it is uncertain just how much more. (You can read more about APOE-2, -3, and -4 in chapter 3 under "Do You Want to Know?") Deterministic genes guarantee that the individual will develop the disease. So far scientists have found rare genes that directly cause Alzheimer's in only a few hundred extended families around the world. Alzheimer's disease caused by deterministic genes is called familial Alzheimer's disease and it accounts for less than 5 percent of all cases.

Here's some interesting recent information about alcohol use and the APOE-4 gene. Studies show that people who have at least one APOE-4 allele have a significantly increased risk of dementia if they consume seven or more drinks per week. In people who do not have the APOE-4 allele, drinking lots of alcohol, even 14 or more drinks per week, is not associated with an increased risk of dementia.

Yet another recent development in the area of genetics and Alzheimer's was uncovered by investigators at Duke University Medical Center. In July 2009, scientists reported what they believe is a gene that is highly predictive of a person's risk of developing Alzheimer's and the approximate age at which the condition will become apparent. The gene has been named TOMM40, and it has mutations that can involve a large number of copies of certain DNA materials in some people. These individuals develop Alzheimer's disease seven years sooner than people who do not have the extra copies.

Now, here are some risk factors over which you have some control.

- **High cholesterol and/or high blood pressure** are both risk factors for heart disease and stroke, but evidence indicates that they increase the likelihood of developing Alzheimer's as well. For example, a large Finnish study of 1,449 people who had high cholesterol and blood pressure found that having these risk factors was more strongly linked to development of Alzheimer's than was carrying the APOE-4 gene. People who had the APOE-4 gene were twice as likely to get Alzheimer's than those without the gene, but among APOE-4 carriers who also had high blood pressure, they were five times more likely to develop Alzheimer's. Among people who also had high cholesterol, the risk for Alzheimer's rose to eight times greater than those without APOE-4.

- **Environmental toxin** exposure is under investigation. For many years, some experts have claimed that aluminum plays a role in the disease. Exposure to aluminum can come from use of aluminum cookware, drinking water, tea, beer, and toothpaste. At this point most experts are not urging people to throw away their aluminum pots, but some people feel more secure in doing so. The potential impact of aluminum or other environmental toxins is still unknown.

- **Educational level** seems to have a role, and research suggests that the more years of formal education people have, the less likely they are to develop Alzheimer's. Experts suggest that longer education may produce stronger and more dense synapses, which could provide some protection against the brain changes associated with Alzheimer's.

- **Diet** increasingly seems to have a role in the development of Alzheimer's disease. Overall, a diet high in fat and sugar and consisting of large amounts of processed and red meats is more conducive to development of Alzheimer's disease than a low-fat, antioxidant-rich diet. (See chapter 4 on prevention for more on diet.)

- **Head trauma** suffered earlier in life appears to be a risk factor for Alzheimer's disease. A history of head injury is clearly a risk factor among people who have the APOE-4 gene.

- **Stress** contributes to the death of brain cells, so it is to your benefit to reduce and manage stress. The hippocampus loses about 6 percent of its cells every decade after age 45, so anything that contributes to that decline is not good for memory.

- **Alcohol use.** When it comes to alcohol and the risk of memory loss and dementia, amount really matters. In a study published in the *Journal of the American Medical Association,* researchers looked at data from 373 people age 65 and older who had dementia and 373 of the same age who did not. They discovered that people who drank 14 or more drinks of alcohol per week had an increased risk of developing dementia. (One drink is defined as 12 ounces of beer, six ounces of wine, or a shot of liquor.) This finding was similar to those seen in previous large studies. They also found, however, that people who had one to six drinks of alcohol per week were 54 percent less likely to develop dementia than people who never drank alcohol. Individuals who drank less than once a week or who had seven to 13 drinks per week also had a reduced risk of dementia, but the investigators were less clear about this relationship.

- **Low estrogen levels** associated with early menopause or hysterectomy may be a risk factor for Alzheimer's disease and dementia. Why? Because estrogen has a protective effect against the development of dementia, and a sharp decline in estrogen levels due to early menopause or hysterectomy is associated with memory problems. We discuss the association between estrogen and memory loss in chapter 4 on prevention.

- **Living alone** has recently been noted as a risk factor for Alzheimer's disease and dementia. A Finnish study published in July 2009 reported that middle-aged people who live alone have twice the risk of developing dementia and Alzheimer's disease in later life compared with married or cohabitating people. People who are widowed or divorced in midlife have three times the risk. This was the first study to focus on the effect of midlife marital status and the risk of dementia. A total of 2,000 men and women were evaluated.

- **Post-traumatic stress disorder (PTSD),** which is common among veterans returning from combat, is associated with reduced cognitive function and an increased risk of dementia. A recent study (2009) conducted by researchers at the University of California, San Francisco, studied 181,093 veterans aged 55 years and older who did not have dementia. At the beginning of the study, a total of 53,155 veterans had a diagnosis of PTSD and 127,938 did not. After tracking the veterans for seven years, the researchers found that those who had PTSD developed new cases of dementia at a rate of 10.6 percent, while those without PTSD had a rate of 6.6 percent.

## Other Types of Dementia

Although Alzheimer's disease makes up about 60 to 65 percent of all cases of dementia, the remaining 35 to 40 percent are mostly rare types of the disease. The most common among this group is vascular dementia, which makes up about 15 percent of all dementias. Vascular dementia is an irreversible form that occurs when the blood flow to the brain is interrupted, causing strokes. Some people who have vascular dementia experience symptoms of stroke such as paralysis on one side of the body, vision problems, and trouble with speech, but others have no symptoms at all. Health-care practitioners can use imaging techniques to distinguish between Alzheimer's disease and vascular dementia.

When abnormal amounts of a protein called Lewy bodies accumulate in nerve cells and destroy them, an individual is diagnosed with Lewy body dementia. Lewy body dementia is more likely to affect attention, thinking, and concentration than memory and language. People who have Lewy body dementia also experience symptoms typical of Parkinson's disease, such as muscle rigidity and tremors.

Several forms of dementia are associated with damage to the front of the brain in the frontal lobe region. One of the most common types of frontal lobe dementia is Pick's disease. This form of dementia usually involves personality and behavior changes before it affects memory and language. People with Pick's disease typically display aggression, rudeness, a lack of inhibition, and inappropriate behavior in public. It affects people of any age but mostly appears between the ages of 40 and 65.

## THE BOTTOM LINE

Memory loss can be attributed to many different factors and conditions, as we demonstrated in this chapter. If you or your loved one has signs and symptoms of Alzheimer's disease, it is time to take the next step, undergoing testing to determine the cause. That's the task we take up in the next chapter on how Alzheimer's disease is diagnosed.

# CHAPTER 3

How Is Alzheimer's Disease Diagnosed?

Some of the most exciting and innovative research in Alzheimer's disease is being done in the areas of screening and diagnosis. Even though there is no cure for Alzheimer's disease at this time, a great many scientists are working on ways to identify, prevent, and treat the disease, and so we are hopeful breakthroughs will occur. In the meantime, if you or a loved one has signs and symptoms of Alzheimer's disease, it is important to seek a doctor's diagnosis as soon as possible so you can know the cause of memory problems and other symptoms and how to take care of them.

With that in mind, we will begin this chapter with the first step in a screening/diagnostic process: finding a knowledgeable doctor. From there we will explore the various approaches to screening and diagnosis of mild cognitive impairment and Alzheimer's disease at your disposal.

## FINDING A KNOWLEDGEABLE HEALTH-CARE PROFESSIONAL

When Bonnie began to notice that her husband was increasingly forgetting names, putting household items in odd places, and showing other symptoms of Alzheimer's disease, she decided they needed to get a professional evaluation. Like many people, however, Bonnie didn't know where to turn.

"We have a primary care doctor, but I really wasn't pleased with him, and I wanted someone who had experience working with older people. I didn't want to talk to my family about it, because I didn't want them to know my suspicions. One of my coworkers has a mother who has Alzheimer's, so I asked her for a recommendation, and we were pleased with our choice."

When looking for a health-care practitioner to help you with your concerns about memory loss and/or Alzheimer's disease, you need a doctor you feel comfortable with. Although no single type of doctor specializes in Alzheimer's disease, there are several specialties that are very knowledgeable about the disease. Many people begin with their primary care physician, but if you do not have one or want to approach another professional, ask for a recommendation from a hospital or trusted family member or friend, or contact your local Alzheimer's Association for help. Primary care physicians often oversee the diagnostic process and may provide treatment themselves, and in many cases they refer patients to a specialist. If you believe you need to consult a specialist and your primary care doctor has not offered a referral, ask for one. Not all specialists are available in every city and town. Here is an explanation of those you can consider.

- **Geriatric psychiatrist**. Physicians who specialize in emotional, mental, and behavioral disorders that commonly affect older adults. Geriatric psychiatrists can prescribe medications.

- **Geriatrician**. Physicians who specialize in the medical conditions that are common among older adults. There is a shortage of geriatricians in the United States. They can serve as primary physicians for older adults.

- **Geriatric nurse practitioner**. These are registered nurses who must have a master's degree and certification through the American Nurses Credentialing Center. They are typically well trained in the behavioral and medication issues related to Alzheimer's.

- **Gerontologist**. These specialists have a masters or doctoral degree in gerontology and can provide nonmedical services to older adults, such as caregiver education and support groups for people who have Alzheimer's disease. Gerontologists are not medical professionals, but they can provide essential support services.

- **Geropsychologist**. The services provided by geropsychologists include psychological testing and therapy related to behavior management, grief and loss, caregiving, and coping mechanisms. Geropsychologists must have a doctorate in psychology and have completed an intensive internship.

- **Neurologist**. These physicians specialize in diseases of the nervous system, including Alzheimer's, Parkinson's, and stroke. Not all neurologists have specific experience working with older adults, however.

- **Neuropsychologist**. Individuals in this specialty can perform neuropsychological testing to identify the impairments associated with Alzheimer's disease, stroke, and other neurological conditions. Neuropsychologists must have a doctorate in psychology and have completed an intensive internship in neuropsychology.

## HOW ALZHEIMER'S DISEASE IS DIAGNOSED

No one test can prove that a person has Alzheimer's disease. In fact, physicians typically need to conduct multiple physical and neurological tests not only to rule out other causes for the patient's symptoms but also to be as accurate as possible. A skilled diagnostician can diagnose Alzheimer's with about 95 percent accuracy. To achieve that level of assurance, practitioners typically conduct selected methods and tests from the list we give below. You may need to go to more than one doctor or facility to undergo all of the tests you need.

- **Patient history**. The information collected by your doctor will include past and current health issues. The items typically covered include information about the main problem, any difficulties concerning daily living activities, information about any other symptoms, history of illnesses and surgeries, medications being taken, family history, psychosocial history (e.g., living conditions, employment, marital status), and mental state. You can help your physician with this part of the evaluation process by being prepared with answers to questions typically asked. See the list under the heading "Questions for the Patient and the Family" on page 43 as a guide.

- **Mini–Mental State Examination (MMSE).** This is a very brief test that can help a physician test a person's attention span, memory, counting skills, and problem-solving skills, and provide some insight into whether parts of the brain may be damaged.

- **Neuropsychological testing.** This is a series of tests that can take two to four hours to complete. The tests are designed to evaluate the relationship between the brain and behavior. This testing process is usually used when patients are having serious problems with memory, understanding language, concentration, remembering words and names, and visual-spatial issues. Neuropsychological testing is preceded by a comprehensive interview with the patient, and then the tests are administered to assess memory, language, the ability to reason, plan, and modify behavior, and an assessment of emotional stability and personality. The clinicians compare skill levels of people who may have Alzheimer's with those of people at the same age and education level. The results of these tests can indicate whether a person can still function independently or if he or she will soon need supervision or another, safer environment. You can see a list of some of the tests under the heading "Neuropsychological Tests" (page 45).

- **Physical examination.** This process allows the doctor to evaluate the patient's overall condition and to determine whether any action is necessary for any medical problems.

- **Chest X-ray**. This test may be ordered if the doctor suspects there may be a condition inside the chest that is causing symptoms similar to those of Alzheimer's disease.

- **Blood tests**. Various tests can be done to look for abnormalities associated with different disorders, such as a vitamin $B_{12}$ deficiency (associated with memory loss) or a thyroid problem. Blood tests can also be used to identify a specific gene that is a risk factor for Alzheimer's disease.

- **Urinalysis**. A urine sample may reveal abnormalities that may be causing symptoms similar to those of Alzheimer's disease.

- **Computed tomography (CT) scan**. This technique uses multiple X-rays taken at different angles to create a series of images. CT scans can show certain changes in the brain that are characteristic of Alzheimer's disease.

- **Magnetic resonance imaging (MRI)**. An MRI uses a large magnet, radio waves, and a computer to produce images of structural and functional changes in the brain that are associated with Alzheimer's disease.

- **Electroencephalography (EEG)**. This technique measures brain function by analyzing the electrical signals produced by the brain. Special electrodes applied to the scalp pick up these messages.

- **Positron emission tomography (PET)** scan. This is a three-dimensional imaging technique that allows physicians to examine the internal organs and determine how they are functioning. PET imaging is capable of showing areas of the brain and thus is useful in evaluating brain disorders like Alzheimer's. PET scans can help differentiate Alzheimer's disease from other dementias, and it can also show the difference in brain activity between a healthy brain and one affected by Alzheimer's disease.

- **Single photon emission computed tomography (SPECT) scan**. This imaging technique produces clear, three-dimensional images of major organs with the help of an injected radioactive substance. The substance emits energy that can be detected by a special camera, which takes pictures of blood flow in the brain. This makes it useful in evaluating brain function and abnormalities characteristic of Alzheimer's disease.

## QUESTIONS FOR THE PATIENT AND THE FAMILY

You can help your doctor, yourself, and your loved one by taking time to write down the answers to the following questions and bringing them with you to your office visit. Be honest and thorough: Sometimes seemingly unimportant information provides insight.

- What symptoms have you noticed? For example, misplacing items, putting objects in inappropriate places (e.g., placing shoes in the refrigerator),

trouble remembering how to do routine tasks,
difficulty remembering names of acquaintances.

• When did these symptoms first appear?

• Have these symptoms changed over time, and
how?

• Do these symptoms interfere or disrupt daily activities? For example, has the ability to drive been
compromised? Do the symptoms affect how the
person performs at work or at other activities such
as volunteer projects? Does the individual turn on
the water and forget that it's on?

• Has the individual ever suffered a head injury
and/or an injury that involved a loss of consciousness? This may include an automobile accident,
sports injury, or fall.

• Does the person have any current medical problems?

• Has the individual had any medical or surgical
procedures in the past?

• What medications (prescription and over-the-
counter) and supplements does the person take
regularly and infrequently? We suggest you bring
all medication and supplement containers with
you so the doctor can see the actual items and the
dosages.

• Does the person drink alcohol and/or is there a
history of alcohol abuse?

## Neuropsychological Tests

- **Mini–Mental State Exam (MMSE)**. This test can detect problems with place and time orientation, object registration, recall, abstract thinking, verbal and written cognition, and constructional abilities. It consists of 30 items, and each item is given one point. A score of less than 24 indicates early to mild dementia.

- **ADAS-Cog (Alzheimer's Disease Assessment Scale-Cognitive)**. This is an 11-part test that takes 30 minutes to complete and is considered to be more thorough than the MMSE. The ADAS-Cog focuses on language, memory skills, executive functioning (ability to make decisions, plan, and perform daily tasks), and orientation (knowing who and where you are).

- **Behavioral Pathology in Alzheimer's Disease Rating Scale (BEHAVE-AD)**. This test rates behavioral symptoms such as physical and verbal aggression and hyperactivity. In addition to diagnosis, some clinicians use it to see how well medications are working to manage behavioral problems.

- **Blessed Test**. This test takes only 10 minutes to complete and assesses memory, attention, concentration, and the ability to complete activities of daily living. Although this is one of the oldest tests, it is still used quite often.

- **CANTAB (Cambridge Neuropsychological Test Automated Battery)**. This battery includes

13 related tests of memory, attention, and the ability to make decisions, plan, and solve complex problems. Individuals use a touch-sensitive computer screen to register their answers. CANTAB is sensitive to early signs of Alzheimer's disease.

• **Clock Drawing Test**. Individuals are asked to draw the face of a clock, place all the numbers, and then show a certain time. This test assesses problems with the ability to perceive objects correctly and the relationship between objects. It is often used along with other neuropsychological tests.

• **Cognistat (Neurobehavioral Cognitive Status Examination)**. This test takes 10 to 30 minutes, depending on the person's level of cognitive impairment. Cognistat assesses intellectual functioning in language, construction (ability to copy or assemble items in a two- or three-dimensional space), memory, calculations, and reasoning/judgment.

• **Dementia Rating Scale-2 (DRS-2)**. This test measures cognitive impairment in five areas: attention, initiation/perseveration (ability to start or stop doing a task), construction, memory, and conceptualization (ability to interpret what you see, hear, etc.).

• **Neuropsychiatric Inventory (NPI)**. Twelve behavioral problems are assessed during this test: agitation, anxiety, apathy, delusions, hallucinations, euphoria (extreme happiness), dysphoria (opposite of euphoria), eating problems, loss of inhibition, irritability, irregular motor behavior (e.g., trembling or shaking of the hands or other body part), and sleeping disturbances.

- **Rey Auditory Verbal Learning Test (RAVLT)**. This test takes about 10 to 15 minutes to administer and consists of two word lists, which individuals are asked to recall on seven different occasions. It measures immediate memory, effects of interference, efficiency of learning, and recall following short and long delays.

## ADVANCES IN THE DIAGNOSIS OF ALZHEIMER'S DISEASE

Although we have just noted the many different tests health-care practitioners can take to help in the diagnosis of Alzheimer's disease, there are other cutting-edge and/or experimental approaches that are or may soon be available. Ask your doctor about one or more of these and other diagnostic advances, as there are new techniques being developed all the time.

- At the 2009 International Conference on Alzheimer's Disease in Vienna, a group of researchers reported that changes in the brain measured using MRI and PET scans, when combined with memory tests and identification of certain proteins in body fluids, may result in earlier and more accurate diagnosis of Alzheimer's. More specifically, the scientists found that detecting Alzheimer's-related proteins (total tau, phosphorylated tau, and beta-amyloid) in the cerebrospinal fluid, along with MRI measurements of the left and right hippocampus and several other brain areas, plus the results of standard memory, learning, and brain function tests (i.e., the Rey Auditory Verbal Learning Test and the ADAS) are helpful in correctly identifying healthy people versus those with Alzheimer's, and people who have mild cognitive impairment who will progress to Alzheimer's. Identification of the APOE-4 allele can provide additional help.

- In June 2009, a study reported that it is now possible to identify which people have a high risk of developing Alzheimer's disease by identifying certain substances in the cerebrospinal fluid.

- A procedure called volumetric MRI (magnetic resonance imaging) is helpful in predicting the progression of mild cognitive impairment to Alzheimer's disease. The study was done by experts at the University of California, San Diego School of Medicine. Volumetric MRI can measure the amount of atrophy in the brain, specifically in the sites related to memory. The procedure can be easily used in clinics.

- While most of the new diagnostic techniques for Alzheimer's disease involve some type of expensive imaging, researchers in Canada developed a technique called near-infrared biospectroscopy, which identifies changes in the blood plasma of Alzheimer's patients. This approach can detect changes very soon after onset of the disease, and possibly even sooner. Biospectroscopy is a technique that uses light or other forms of energy to detect the composition of substances because different substances reflect or emit light at specific, detectable wavelengths. The Canadian researchers applied the technique to blood plasma samples taken from patients who had early Alzheimer's dementia or mild cognitive impairment, as well as from healthy elderly volunteers. They were able to correctly distinguish the Alzheimer's patients from the healthy controls with 80 percent sensitivity (correctly identified patients with disease) and 77 percent specificity (correctly identified individuals without disease). Many of the subjects who had mild cognitive impairment tested positively with the Alzheimer's patients, which suggested to the researchers that the test may be helpful in detecting Alzheimer's disease before patients have noticeable symptoms.

## DO YOU WANT TO KNOW?

Let's say you're 43 years old and you don't have any signs or symptoms of Alzheimer's disease, but your grandfather died of the disease and your mother has just been diagnosed at age 70. Do you have the right to know if you have the genes that put you at high risk for the disease? Do you *want* to know?

In a study conducted at Boston University School of Medicine, researchers examined the impact of telling the adult children of patients who have Alzheimer's disease what their genetic risk was for getting the disease themselves. The study was quite appropriately called the REVEAL Study, and the results were published in the July 16, 2009, issue of the *New England Journal of Medicine*. They showed that distress related to the test was reduced among participants who learned that they were not carriers of APOE-4, and that it was high only temporarily among participants who learned they were APOE-4 positive. The study also showed that people who were very distressed before undergoing genetic testing were more likely to have emotional difficulties after learning the test results.

Although there is a blood test designed to identify which form of APOE a person has, it is not yet possible to reliably predict who will and who will not develop Alzheimer's disease (see below). For now, APOE testing is largely reserved for research settings to identify study participants who may be at increased risk for developing Alzheimer's. For people who are at high risk of developing early-onset Alzheimer's disease, however, genetic testing is more readily available.

Here is what the experts know about the three different forms of APOE (APOE-2, -3, and -4) and the chances of people in the general population getting Alzheimer's disease.

- About 60 percent of people inherit two APOE-3 genes, which does not increase their risk of developing Alzheimer's disease. Therefore about half of these individuals will develop the disease by age 80 to 85.

- About 25 percent of people inherit one copy of APOE-4, which increases their risk of developing Alzheimer's disease by three times in men and four times in women.

- About 2 percent of people inherit two copies of APOE-4, which increases their risk of getting Alzheimer's disease by about fifteen times compared with people who have no APOE-4 gene.

- About 16 percent of people inherit the APOE-2 gene, and 11 percent have one APOE-2 and one APOE-3 gene. These individuals are partially protected against getting the disease because their risk of developing Alzheimer's does not reach 50 percent until their late nineties. Only 0.5 percent of people inherit two copies of the APOE-2 gene, and they have a very low risk of getting the disease.

## THE BOTTOM LINE

Although there is no single test to identify Alzheimer's disease with 100 percent accuracy, the battery of diagnostic tools that doctors have at their disposal, when applied judiciously, can provide an accurate diagnosis in about 95 percent of cases. That 5-percent gap may be closed someday soon, as improved technologies and techniques are developed. Naturally, getting a diagnosis is just the beginning of the journey, and so the next part of this book talks about what you and your loved ones can do to make that journey as loving and healthy as possible.

# PART II

**Everything You Need to Know About Prevention and Treatment**

# CHAPTER 4

How to Prevent Alzheimer's Disease

There is no cure for Alzheimer's disease . . . yet! But the sheer volume of research being done on the causes, diagnosis, and treatment of Alzheimer's disease offers hope to everyone who is touched by the disease—and nearly everyone is, either directly or indirectly.

That's why in this chapter we explore the steps you can take to help prevent memory loss and Alzheimer's disease. An added bonus of these steps and recommendations is that they also may benefit those who already have early Alzheimer's disease by improving their quality of life and in some cases, may even help preserve memory longer. One recommendation we do not discuss at length in this chapter is a very popular and effective one—brain exercises. This technique is so important as both a preventive and treatment approach for memory loss and Alzheimer's disease that we have dedicated all of chapter 9 to it.

As for the recommendations we offer in this chapter, you may recognize most of them as the same suggestions offered to people to prevent cardiovascular and cerebrovascular disease.

Yes, it's true that there is a close association between

memory loss and Alzheimer's disease, and heart disease and stroke. If this is news to you, you are not alone.

In July 2009, the results of an online survey conducted by researchers at the University of Connecticut were published in *Alzheimers and Dementia*. The researchers found that 64 percent of the people questioned (the participants had a mean age of 50 and were well-educated) did not know there was an association between Alzheimer's and obesity or high blood pressure, both of which are significant risk factors for heart disease. Sixty-six percent did not know that high stress is a risk factor for dementia, and 34 percent did not know that physical exercise can protect against the disease. Most (94 percent) of the people surveyed, however, did know that Alzheimer's disease is not part of normal aging and is not completely based on genetics.

So, consider this chapter a bonus: You can significantly improve your chances of preventing Alzheimer's disease *and* help keep your heart and brain healthy if you follow the lifestyle suggestions in this chapter.

## WHAT'S SO GREAT ABOUT EXERCISE?

For people who have early Alzheimer's disease, the results of a study published in July 2008 may be just what the doctor ordered when it comes to exercise. The researchers found that individuals who had early Alzheimer's disease and who were less physically fit had four times more brain shrinkage than healthy older adults who were more physically fit.

To arrive at their conclusion, the researchers tested the participants on treadmills to assess their physical activity level, administered mental assessments, and used MRIs to examine their brains. The investigators believe that regular exercise has the potential to reduce the amount of brain volume lost and thus preserve brain function longer in people who have early Alzheimer's disease.

Study after study has shown that physical exercise—and specifically aerobic exercise such as brisk walking, jogging, dancing, and tennis—improves the ability to think, remember, and concentrate. A significant report was released in May 2009 by the National Institute on Aging, which is part of the National Institutes of Health. In it, researchers noted that "evidence is accumulating that exercise has profound benefits for brain function," and that "physical activity improves learning and memory in humans" and "might prevent or delay loss of cognitive function with aging or neurodegenerative disease" such as Alzheimer's.

During the Alzheimer's Association 2009 International Conference on Alzheimer's Disease in Vienna, researchers reported on the newest findings on exercise and Alzheimer's. In the Health, Aging, and Body Composition Study, which included 3,075 people ages 70 to 79, the investigators assessed physical activity and cognitive function at the beginning of the study and again after two, four, and seven years. They found that older adults who were sedentary throughout the study had the lowest levels of cognitive function and the fastest rate of cognitive decline.

Some research has even gone so far as to show that people who carry APOE-4 could get more benefit from maintaining an active lifestyle than those who do not have this allele. In one such study, for example, older women who had APOE-4 and who participated in aerobic exercise performed better on auditory, spatial, and visual learning tasks than women who were not carriers.

## Enough Talk, Time for Action

You have probably heard all the excuses people give as to why they can't exercise, and not having enough time is near if not at the top of the list. You may have used some of the excuses yourself. But with just minimal planning, you can make subtle changes in your lifestyle that can open up time for regular exercise: about 30 minutes of aerobic activity four to five times per week.

## Exercise Guidelines

• Include a few minutes of gentle warm-up and cool-down activity with each exercise session. Some experts recommend 15 minutes of each, but given that many people are pressed for time, this may not be possible. Even five minutes of warm-up and cool-down are helpful.

• Choose activities that you enjoy. Your exercise experiences can be more fun if you try different activities on alternate days. For example, a brisk walk before breakfast three days a week, alternated with an aerobic class or time on a stationary bike on two days.

• Share your exercise experience with a friend or group. You may be surprised how fast your 45-minute walk passes by if you are walking and talking with a friend. Consider joining an aerobic team activity, such as tennis, badminton, or pickleball, once or twice a week.

• Make sure you are properly dressed and protected for the activity of your choice. This precaution includes wearing good walking or jogging shoes and a helmet if you ride a bicycle.

- Find ways to include more physical activity into your daily life. Take the stairs instead of the elevator, walk to the local store, rake leaves instead of blowing them, and try your hand at gardening.

- Weight and resistance training not only increases muscle mass, it can also help maintain memory. If you add two to three strength exercise sessions to your daily aerobic routine, you may reduce your risk of Alzheimer's by 50 percent if you are older than 65.

The bottom line is, keep moving to help keep your memory.

## NONSTEROIDAL ANTI-INFLAMMATORY DRUGS

Is it possible that the ibuprofen or naproxen you take for your tension headache could also help protect you against Alzheimer's disease? Over the years, various studies have evaluated the use of these and other nonsteroidal anti-inflammatory drugs (NSAIDs) as a preventive measure against development of Alzheimer's disease, and the results have not always agreed. In one study conducted by the National Institutes of Health, the researchers found that people who took ibuprofen for two years had half the risk of developing Alzheimer's disease as people who did not take the drug.

The Alzheimer's Disease Anti-inflammatory Prevention Trial (ADAPT) was designed to determine whether nonsteroidal anti-inflammatory drugs can prevent or delay the onset of Alzheimer's disease. The more than 2,600 participants were age 70 or older and had a family history of Alzheimer-like dementia. They were randomly assigned to take 200 mg naproxen, 200 mg celecoxib (Celebrex), or a placebo twice daily. The study was suspended early because use of celecoxib was associated with an increased risk of heart attacks and stroke.

Once the study was halted, the researchers continued to follow the study participants. An average of two years after the study was stopped, the investigators noted that naproxen reduced the risk of developing Alzheimer's disease by two-thirds. Researchers noted that it appears that NSAIDs harm people who already have signs and symptoms of dementia, but for people who have healthy brains, NSAIDs seem to offer some protection against Alzheimer's disease.

Should you take naproxen to protect yourself and your loved ones against Alzheimer's disease? Experts emphasize that they need more information on the effectiveness of these drugs. They also mention that long-term use of NSAIDs is associated with stomach bleeding and an increased risk of cardiovascular disease.

Therefore, if you are already taking NSAIDs for another condition, you could be reducing your risk of developing Alzheimer's disease. But if you do not already take NSAIDs, it is best to wait until further research uncovers more about the impact of these drugs on Alzheimer's disease and overall health. (You can read more about NSAIDs and Alzheimer's disease on page 81.)

## ACE INHIBITORS

A class of medication called ACE (angiotensin-converting enzyme) inhibitors, which are used to treat high blood pressure, appear to help protect older adults against memory loss and other cognitive problems. The research findings were published in July 2009 by investigators at Wake Forest University School of Medicine. The authors of the study found that ACE inhibitors may reduce inflammation that could contribute to the development of Alzheimer's disease.

Although the findings are preliminary at this point, they do make us wonder whether other blood pressure drugs could be helpful as well. The investigators noted that they believe blood pressure medications differ when it comes to reducing the risk of dementia in people who have high blood pressure. In fact, they note that not all ACE inhibitors are equally effective. Some ACE inhibitors can cross the blood-brain barrier, a special network of blood vessels that protect the brain from infiltration by harmful substances. These ACE inhibitors are known as "centrally acting" because they can cross the barrier. Centrally acting ACE inhibitors include captropril (Capoten), fosinopril (Monopril), lisinopril (Prinivil, Zestri), perindopril (Accon), ramipril (Altace), and trandolapril (Mavik).

The study evaluated 1,074 patients who had high blood pressure but did not have dementia at the start of the study. All participants were treated with either centrally active or non–centrally active ACE inhibitors. The investigators observed a significant cognitive benefit among participants who were taking centrally active ACE inhibitors: These patients had an average 65 percent less cognitive decline per year taking the drugs compared to patients who took other blood pressure medications.

The same was not true for non–centrally active ACE inhibitors. In fact, the researchers discovered that patients who took the ACE inhibitors that did not cross the blood-brain barrier had a 73 percent greater risk of developing dementia than patients who were taking other medications for high blood pressure. Thus the scientists suggest that when doctors are considering giving patients an ACE inhibitor, it may be best to prescribe one that can get into the brain.

## EAT, DRINK, AND HAVE MEMORY

Can you eat to protect your memory and perhaps prevent Alzheimer's disease? A growing amount of evidence says yes. For example, at the 2009 International Conference on Alzheimer's Disease, new research indicated that the Dietary Approaches to Stop Hypertension (DASH) eating plan may reduce age-related cognitive decline. The DASH eating plan (see below, "Eating the DASH Way") has been proven to lower blood pressure, and high blood pressure is a risk factor for Alzheimer's disease and other dementias.

To help prove the point, a recent study (Cache County Study on Memory, Health and Aging) examined the association between how closely people followed the DASH diet and their risk of cognitive decline and dementia. The study included 3,831 participants age 65 years or older and covered an 11-year period. Cognitive function was evaluated four times over the study period. The researchers found that participants who had the highest DASH scores also had the highest cognitive functioning scores. They also found that of the nine food-group/nutrient components (fruit, vegetables, nut/legumes, whole grains, low-fat dairy, sodium, sweets, non-fish meat, and fish), the foods that offered the most benefits for cognition in later life were whole grains, vegetables, low-fat dairy, and nuts.

## EATING THE DASH WAY

| Food Group | Servings on 2,000 Calorie Diet |
|---|---|
| Grains and grain products | 7–8 |
| Fruits | 4–5 |
| Vegetables | 4–5 |
| Low and nonfat dairy | 2–3 |
| Lean meat, fish, poultry | 2 or less |

Nuts, seeds, and legumes     4–5/week
Fats and sweets     limited

---

### How Big Is a Serving?

**Grains and Grain Products:** 1 slice of bread, ½ cup cooked cereal, rice, or pasta, or 1 ounce of ready-to-eat cereal

**Vegetables:** ½ cup cooked or chopped raw vegetables, ¾ cup vegetable juice, or 1 cup raw leafy vegetables

**Fruits:** 1 apple, banana, or orange, ¾ cup fruit juice, or ½ cup chopped, cooked, or canned fruit

**Meat, Poultry, Fish, Dry Beans, Eggs, Nuts:** 2 to 3 ounces of cooked meat, poultry, or fish; eating ½ cup cooked beans, 1 egg, or 2 tablespoons nut butter equals one ounce of meat

**Dairy:** 1 cup milk, 1½ to 2 ounces of cheese, or 1 cup yogurt

---

### A Few Words about Fat

Research has shown that a low-fat diet, and one that includes "good" fat, benefits the brain. The question is, "What is low and good?"

Depending on which expert you talk to, the definition of a "low fat" diet ranges from less than 10 to 30 percent of total caloric intake daily. Studies done using various amounts within that range have shown positive results when it comes to reducing the risk of developing Alzheimer's disease.

For example, Dean Ornish, M.D., a practicing physician

and author of *Eat More, Weigh Less,* has been very successful in improving and even reversing heart disease in patients. His dietary plan involves less than 10 percent of calories from fat and is considered a very low-fat diet. In a Case Western Reserve University study, investigators found that young and middle-aged adults who consumed a diet that contained 20 percent fat significantly reduced their risk of developing Alzheimer's. A 2002 study reported that people who ate the most calories and fat had twice the risk of developing Alzheimer's disease than people who consumed a lower-calorie, lower-fat diet.

You also should not forget that a low-fat diet has other benefits, such as helping with weight loss and keeping cholesterol levels down. Both excess weight and body fat, as well as high cholesterol, are risk factors for transient ischemic attacks and strokes, which can hinder blood flow in the brain and cause memory problems and increase the risk for Alzheimer's disease.

Now let's consider "good" fat. Good fats promote brain health and function, as well as overall health. Omega-3 fatty acids, a type of polyunsaturated fat that is found in certain cold-water fish (e.g., tuna, herring, salmon), olive oil, canola oil, flaxseed oil, green leafy vegetables, nuts, and avocados, comprise a good fat. (We discuss omega-3 fatty acids in more detail below.) Monounsaturated fat also is a good fat because it can help reduce cholesterol and the risk of Alzheimer's, stroke, and heart disease. This fat is found primarily in vegetable oils such as olive, canola, peanut, and sesame oil, as well as avocados and many seeds and nuts.

If there are good fats, then there must be bad ones, and in the bad category are saturated fats, trans fats, and omega-6 fatty acids (a type of polyunsaturated fat). Both saturated fat and omega-6 fatty acids are found in meat and other animal foods (e.g., cheese, milk, butter), as well as processed foods and fried foods. Trans fats are found in some margarines and in some vegetable oils and many fried and processed foods (e.g., French fries, frozen dinners, snack foods, crackers, cookies, baked goods).

Thus if you follow a low-fat diet and the fats in your diet are mostly omega-3 fatty acids and monounsaturated fats, then you are taking positive steps to prevent memory loss and Alzheimer's disease.

## Omega-3 Fatty Acids

There's something fishy about it—but in this case that's sometimes a good thing. At the Alzheimer's Association 2009 International Conference on Alzheimer's Disease, one of the featured studies involved giving omega-3 fatty acid supplements or a placebo to 485 healthy adults age 55 and older who had complaints of only mild memory problems. The researchers found that the participants who took 900 mg of docosahexanoic acid (DHA) daily for six months had nearly double the reduction in mistakes on a test that measures learning and memory skills, compared with people who took a placebo.

According to one of the study's authors, the benefits offered by the omega-3 supplements are roughly equal to having the learning and memory capabilities of someone three years younger. The not-so-great news? Another study that administered 2 grams daily of DHA to people who had mild to moderate Alzheimer's disease found that the supplements did not slow the progression of Alzheimer's. Therefore DHA appears to be helpful in preventing but not in treating memory loss.

## Other Dietary Factors

In people who have Alzheimer's disease, inflammation and insulin resistance can damage nerve cells and thus impair communication between brain cells. Another dietary factor that increases the risk of Alzheimer's disease is high cholesterol. While the DASH eating plan addresses these risk factors, the following tips can be helpful as well:

- Maintain consistent blood sugar and insulin levels. This can be easy to do if you eat small meals throughout the day and avoid refined and processed foods, especially those consisting of white flour and sugars, which can cause your glucose levels to spike. Why is this important? Because the brain's main food source is glucose, and a rapid rise in glucose levels can cause inflammation.

- Make sure you get enough omega-3 fatty acids, as they are proven to enhance brain function. Foods rich in omega-3 fatty acids include some mentioned in the DASH plan, such as cold water fish (e.g., tuna, herring, salmon) and nuts.

- Focus on foods rich in antioxidants, as these substances destroy free radicals, which are cell-damaging molecules. Fruits and vegetables are high in antioxidants, as are many whole grains, legumes, and nuts.

- Green tea, as well as white and oolong teas, have proven to be good for the brain. The recommended "dose" is two to four cups daily.

- Avoid commercial salad dressings and condiments and make your own using olive oil or flax-seed oil, along with vinegars, herbs, spices, and pureed vegetables.

• If you eat poultry, do not eat the skin, and limit your intake to 2 ounces or less daily.

• If you eat meat, trim off all fat, buy the leanest cuts, and limit your intake to 2 ounces or less daily.

• Focus on plant proteins, which do not contain cholesterol and saturated fat. Plant protein foods include soybeans and soybean products (e.g., tofu, soy milk, textured vegetable protein), beans, tempeh, split peas, and lentils.

• Eat foods high in fiber. They can help with weight control and blood sugar levels. The recommended intake of fiber per day is 25 to 30 grams. Foods rich in fiber include oatmeal, fresh fruits and vegetables, beans, lentils, split peas, and whole grain breads and other products.

• Keep sugar intake to a minimum. Excess sugar can be converted by the body into saturated fat, which harms the brain and heart. A high-sugar diet can increase free radical activity and damage brain cells, which contributes to memory problems. The U.S. Dietary Guidelines note that the average person should consume no more than the equivalent of 10 teaspoons of sugar daily. If you drink one can of regular cola, you have just consumed about 11 teaspoons! To calculate how much sugar you are getting, read nutritional labels. Four grams of sugar equals 1 teaspoon of sugar.

• Consider caffeine carefully. On the positive side, caffeine enhances mood, reduces fatigue, increases attention, and boosts energy levels for some people. If you already consume caffeinated beverages (e.g., coffee, tea, hot chocolate) and you do not experience any negative side effects such as insomnia, nervousness, headaches, and stomach irritation, then you can probably continue drinking them. If you don't drink such beverages, there's no reason to start and risk having side effects.

## SLEEP = BETTER MEMORY

Losing sleep can cause a lot more than yawns: It can have a significant impact on brain functioning. The brain requires regular, restful sleep to process, store, and retrieve memories. A recent (2009) study conducted in Belgium, for example, found that sleep promotes memory consolidation, a process by which the brain reorganizes new memories into stable ones. People who were sleep-deprived were much less able to recall memories than those who were not sleep-deprived. The researchers even documented the recollection of memories using magnetic resonance imaging (MRI).

According to Vincent Fortanasce, M.D., neurologist, director of the Fortanasce Neurology Center in Arcadia, California, and author of *The Anti-Alzheimer's Prescription,* sleep is essential to replenish the neurotransmitters dopamine and serotonin, which increase the feelings of self-control and well-being. Dopamine also decreases anxiety.

Too much sleep, however, may be detrimental. A German study published in 2009 followed more than 4,000 older adults and monitored their sleep duration and cognitive abilities. At the 15-year follow-up, the investigators found no relationship between sleeping less than or equal to six hours and up to eight hours and cognitive impairment, but there was cognitive and verbal memory impairment in those who slept nine hours or longer. The bottom line is, get enough sleep, but not too much!

To help you get restful sleep, try these suggestions:

- **Be regular**. If you go to bed and get up at the same time every day, you reinforce your circadian rhythm. It may take you a little time to establish this pattern, but it's worth it.

- **Set the mood**. The bed should be reserved for sleep (and sex), not for other activities that can keep you awake. Taking a hot shower, dimming the lights, adding aromatherapy (lavender is relaxing), and using white noise machines can help set the mood for sleep.

- **Treat sleep apnea**. Research shows that 70 to 80 percent of people who have Alzheimer's disease experience sleep apnea. Cognition can improve with the use of continuous positive airway pressure (CPAP) treatment, which regulates the amount of oxygen available to the brain.

- **Turn off your mind**. If mental chatter is disturbing your ability to sleep, try relaxation methods, such as meditation, reading, listening to soothing music, or deep breathing exercises.

## MANAGE STRESS

According to Dr. Fortanasce, chronic stress can double or quadruple your risk of developing Alzheimer's disease. A major reason for this increased risk is that stress elevates levels of the stress hormone cortisol, which damages nerve cells and accelerates cognitive decline, depression, diabetes, and other attacks on the brain. It's been known for many years that higher levels of stress hormones are seen in people who have early Alzheimer's disease.

More evidence comes from the University of California, Irvine, where researchers found that stress hormones can rapidly increase the formation of the brain lesions that are associated with Alzheimer's disease. They suggest that managing stress could help prevent and significantly slow down progression of the disease.

How can you manage the stress in your life and in that of your loved ones? Here are a few suggestions.

- **Stay connected socially**. It is critically important to socialize and interact with other people on a regular basis. Some older individuals isolate themselves, especially if they have lost a partner or good friend. Establishing a social and support network with neighbors, a church or spiritual group, a volunteer organization, or another community group can provide such a connection.

- **Practice breathing exercises**. Stress has a negative impact on breathing and thus changes the amount of oxygen that reaches the brain. The practice of deep, slow, abdominal breathing can be very powerful and relaxing. You can easily learn how to do such breathing through videos on the Internet or at public libraries, by attending guided group sessions, or from books or articles on the subject.

- **Schedule daily relaxation sessions**. You need to relax more than once a week to keep cortisol levels under control. Make time for yourself every day: schedule a walk, practice tai chi or yoga, go to the library and read in a quiet corner, or watch a funny movie.

• **Cultivate inner peace**. The strong mind-body connection is a powerful one, and some research indicates that personal spiritual pursuits can enhance cognitive functioning, likely by reducing the damaging impact of stress. Spiritual practice can be whatever works for you, be it meditation, religious practice, prayer, or trying new spiritual paths.

## HORMONE REPLACEMENT THERAPY

The question as to whether women should take hormone replacement therapy to help ward off Alzheimer's disease and other dementias is one that brings up a lot of anxiety for many people, and much of that anxiety revolves around the findings of the Women's Health Initiative.

The Women's Health Initiative included more than 4,500 women between the ages of 65 and 80 who were taking horse-derived estrogen and synthetic progesterone in a drug called Prempro. The study was stopped before it was scheduled to end because the researchers found that the hormone replacement therapy was associated with a twofold increase in the prevalence of Alzheimer's disease and other dementias, as well as an increased risk of venous thrombosis, stroke, and breast cancer.

Another risk has been associated with hormone replacement therapy. A new study (July 2009) found that compared with women who have never taken hormone therapy, those who currently take it or who have used it in the past are at increased risk of ovarian cancer. This risk is not affected by how long women have used the therapy, the formulation, estrogen dose, or the type of therapy used.

Yet scientists also know that a decline in estrogen levels, which occurs when women go through menopause or have a hysterectomy that ends her menstrual cycle, is associated with memory loss and problems with concentration and attention. Therefore it seems to make sense to take estrogen to restore the hormone levels and boost the brain. The question now becomes, How can estrogen help memory yet increase the risk of losing it?

Part of the answer may lie in the type of estrogen and progesterone given to women. Rather than horse-derived estrogen and synthetic progesterone, both of which are viewed as foreign by the body, studies show that women respond positively to bioidentical estrogen and progesterone—that is, hormones that mimic those produced by the body. These include soy-based estrogen and micronized progesterone, options women should discuss with their health-care providers when discussing ways to prevent Alzheimer's disease.

## BOOST YOUR BRAIN POWER

More and more today we hear about ways to exercise your brain, enhance your brain cells, and put your neurons to work. That's because studies strongly suggest that people can reduce the risk of developing Alzheimer's disease if they routinely engage in activities that stimulate the mind, such as reading, writing, playing instruments, learning new languages or hobbies, and doing puzzles.

Results of one of the more recent studies was presented at the American Academy of Neurology's 61st Annual Meeting in Seattle in spring 2009. A research team evaluated 197 people between the ages of 70 and 89 who had mild cognitive impairment or diagnosed memory loss and 1,124 people of the same age who had no memory problems. All the participants were questioned about their daily activities over the past year and when they were 50 to 65 years old.

The investigators found that during their later years, individuals who participated in computer activities, did crafts, read books, and played games had a 30 to 50 percent decreased risk of developing memory problems compared with people who did not participate in such activities. One significant negative factor in retaining memory is television: The researchers found that people who watched television for fewer than seven hours a day in later years were 50 percent less likely to develop memory problems than people who watched it for longer than seven hours daily.

Regularly engaging in mentally stimulating activities is a critically important factor in preventing memory loss and helping to prevent dementia. Participating in such mental exercises appears to increase the number of neurons as well as strengthen the connections between them. That's why we have dedicated an entire chapter to "brain exercises" you can do to not only prevent Alzheimer's disease but also slow progress of the disease if you or a loved one is diagnosed with the disease. These exercises will also improve your lifestyle. (See chapter 9.)

## THE BOTTOM LINE

The things you need to do to prevent Alzheimer's disease are related to lifestyle: diet, exercise, stress management, sleep, and judicious use of certain medications and hormones. In the next chapter we discuss alternative and complementary approaches to the prevention and treatment of Alzheimer's disease.

# CHAPTER 5

How to Treat Alzheimer's with Drugs

The drugs currently available to treat Alzheimer's disease and its various symptoms can provide relief and slow progression of the disease, but they do not cure the disease. This may be one of the most difficult facts for people to accept about Alzheimer's disease and dementia. Despite the growing popularity of alternative and complementary medicine, much of Western society depends on—and expects—medications to relieve and cure their ills. When we talk about Alzheimer's disease, however, this expectation cannot be met—yet.

The vast scope of research surrounding the development of more effective treatments and the search for a cure for Alzheimer's disease are hopeful signs that a cure will be found someday. Until then, we have many helpful medications that can be combined with complementary approaches, which we discuss in chapter 6, that can offer people who have Alzheimer's disease and their loved ones a better quality of life.

In this chapter we explore the medications that have been approved for treatment of the cognitive symptoms of Alzheimer's disease, as well as those that are used off-label for this purpose. We also explore the drugs that are often used to manage behavioral and psychiatric symptoms. We suggest you use the information in this chapter, along with that in the next chapter on complementary therapies, when you and your doctor sit down and discuss how to develop a treatment plan.

## TREATING COGNITIVE SYMPTOMS

Currently there are two classes of drugs on the market that have been approved by the U.S. Food and Drug Administration (FDA) to treat cognitive symptoms associated with Alzheimer's disease. These two classes of drugs affect the activity of two different chemicals involved in transporting messages between the neurons in the brain. Fortunately, clinicians can and do often prescribe one medication from each group for their patients, as these drugs can work well together. We will discuss each drug separately below.

### Cholinesterase Inhibitors

Cholinesterase inhibitors are the most commonly prescribed drugs for the treatment of Alzheimer's disease. These drugs work by preventing the breakdown of acetylcholine, a chemical that is essential for learning and memory. Basically, cholinesterase inhibitors help keep acetylcholine levels high so the chemical can continue to support communication among nerve cells. On average, cholinesterase inhibitors can delay worsening of cognitive symptoms for six to 12 months for about 50 percent of patients who use these drugs. Some patients do far better longer on these drugs, but for now there is no way to identify which patients will do so.

There is also some evidence that cholinesterase inhibitors could help people who have mild cognitive impairment. A study published in the June 2009 issue of *Neurology*, for example, found that one of the drugs in this class, donepezil, reduced progression to Alzheimer's disease in patients who had depression and mild cognitive impairment.

**Donepezil.** This cholinesterase inhibitor (Aricept®) is the most commonly prescribed cholinesterase inhibitor for people who have Alzheimer's disease and the only one in this class that has been approved to treat all stages of Alzheimer's disease, from mild to severe. The drug is derived from components of black pepper.

Patients who take donepezil tend to tolerate it relatively well, although there are some side effects associated with its use. In rare cases, severe diarrhea or sedation may occur. More commonly people say they have vivid nightmares, bloating, and a runny nose, any or all of which may occur after patients have reached their maximum effective dose. The typical dosage is one tablet daily (regular or disintegrating type) taken at bedtime, with or without food. Treatment usually begins at 5 mg per day over about four to six weeks, increasing to 10 mg after that time.

**Galantamine.** The FDA has approved galantamine (Razadyne®, formerly called Reminyl) to treat mild to moderate Alzheimer's disease. Galantamine is derived from daffodil bulbs, and along with preventing the breakdown of acetylcholine, it also stimulates nicotinic receptors to release more acetylcholine in the brain. The typical dose is one regular tablet (4 mg) taken twice daily with morning and evening meals, or one extended-release tablet (8 mg) taken once daily with the morning meal. Your doctor may increase the dose if needed. The side effects are similar to those associated with donepezil.

**Rivastigmine.** Like galantamine, rivastigmine (Exelon®) has been approved for treatment of mild to moderate Alzheimer's disease. This drug prevents the breakdown of both acetylcholine and butyrylcholine, a chemical in the brain that is similar to acetylcholine. One advantage of this drug is that it is available in liquid and patch forms, which is helpful for patients who have difficulty swallowing pills.

The typical starting oral dose of rivastigmine is 1.5 mg twice daily taken for a minimum of two weeks. If that dose is well tolerated, your doctor may increase the dose to 3 mg twice daily. The maximum recommended dose is 6 mg taken two times per day. The patch is applied once daily and slowly releases the prescribed amount over 24 hours.

The most common side effects associated with rivastigmine are nausea, diarrhea, and vomiting. People who have heart or lung conditions, seizures, or bladder problems should consult their doctors before using this drug.

**Tacrine.** This drug (Cognex®) was the first one approved for treatment of Alzheimer's disease. Today it has been virtually removed from the market because it provides only modest benefits, it can damage the liver, and it offers no help to people who have the APOE-4 allele. Fortunately the other three drugs in this class are not burdened with these adverse effects.

**Memantine.** Currently, memantine (Namenda®) is in a class by itself as the only drug approved thus far that works by regulating the activity of glutamate. The official name for the drug class is N-methyl-D-aspartate (NMDA) receptor antagonists. Glutamate is a chemical in the brain that also acts as a messenger and is involved in memory and learning. Large amounts of this chemical, however, have toxic effects on the brain. In people who have Alzheimer's disease, their damaged neurons release high levels of glutamate. Memantine protects the brain against overstimulation by glutamate by blocking NDMA receptors and thus helps reduce the damage excessive glutamate can cause.

Memantine, which was approved in October 2003, got the go-ahead by the FDA for treatment of moderate to severe Alzheimer's disease. Like cholinesterase inhibitors, memantine temporarily delays worsening of cognitive symptoms in some people who take the drug, although it works differently than cholinesterase inhibitors. Because these two classes of drugs act in different ways on the brain, people with Alzheimer's disease can often benefit from taking both types of medications. Thus many physicians prescribe memantine along with a cholinesterase inhibitor to treat all stages of Alzheimer's disease, from mild to severe.

That was the case for Hazel, a 75-year-old great-grandmother, who had been experiencing significant memory problems for about one year when her daughter, Bridget, brought her to a neurologist to be tested for Alzheimer's disease. Hazel also had a history of high blood pressure and high cholesterol. Once Hazel was diagnosed with mild Alzheimer's disease, the doctor first prescribed donepezil, and then added memantine after several months, as well as vitamin $B_{12}$ and folic acid, to see if it would help slow progression of the disease. (We discuss use of these supplements in chapter 6.)

Nearly two years after Hazel started treatment, Bridget reported that her mother was still able to continue her favorite activities—reading, knitting, and going to church—at nearly the same level as she had before the diagnosis. Although Bridget realizes that her mother will eventually lose these abilities, they are both grateful for the quality of life she has had while following this treatment course.

Like other people who are prescribed memantine, Hazel started with 5 mg once daily. Her doctor then increased her dose to 5 mg twice daily, then 15 mg daily (one 5-mg and one 10-mg dose), and finally 10 mg twice daily. The minimum recommended time between increases in dose is one week. Memantine can be taken with or without food.

The most common side effects associated with memantine include dizziness (occurs in about 7 percent of patients), constipation (6 percent), and headache (6 percent). Memantine is well tolerated by most patients, but those who have kidney disease, urinary tract problems, epilepsy, or a history of seizures need to consult with their doctor before taking this medication.

## Other Options for Treating Cognitive Symptoms

Several other medications that are not specifically targeted for treatment of cognitive symptoms have demonstrated some benefit in patients who have the disease. Therefore, many physicians include these drugs in their arsenal when determining how to treat their patients. Let's take a look at these options.

**Selegiline.** Although selegiline is perhaps best known as a drug treatment for Parkinson's disease, it also has been found to be beneficial for some patients who have Alzheimer's disease. Selegiline fights Alzheimer's disease on two fronts: As an antioxidant it destroys free radicals (which damage brain cells) and it inhibits the monoamine oxidase (MAO) enzyme, which destroys neurotransmitters in the brain.

In the short term, some research shows that selegiline can delay progression of Alzheimer's disease by as much as seven months. Beyond that, the advantages are uncertain. In a recent study (July 2008) from Japan, however, researchers found that the use of both selegiline and donepezil provided a synergistic effect, with selegiline seeming to enhance the cognitive benefits of donepezil.

Selegiline is available in tablets and capsules. The most

common side effects include insomnia, psychosis, and confusion. Your doctor will prescribe a dose best suited for your needs.

**Nonsteroidal anti-inflammatory drugs.** You may recall that we discussed nonsteroidal anti-inflammatory drugs (NSAIDs) in chapter 4, where we noted that they may be helpful in preventing memory loss and Alzheimer's disease. In addition, some studies also suggest that this class of drugs may be beneficial in the treatment of Alzheimer's disease, while others dispute this claim.

For example, while several studies suggest that longterm use of NSAIDs offer protection against Alzheimer's disease, especially for people who have one or more APOE-4 alleles, others indicate that chronic use of NSAIDs is only helpful in preventing Alzheimer's disease in healthy brains. Once an accumulation of beta-amyloid has started, NSAIDs do not appear to be effective and may even be harmful. An April 2009 study that looked at the use of ibuprofen (400 mg twice daily) in patients who had mild to moderate Alzheimer's disease found that the NSAID was not effective in reducing cognitive decline except in patients who had the APOE-4 allele.

For now, it appears that the jury is still out on the benefits of NSAIDs in the treatment of Alzheimer's disease. We also want to note that use of NSAIDs along with cholinesterase inhibitors should be done with caution, as the combination increases the risk of bleeding of the gastrointestinal tract.

**Statins.** The drugs most commonly prescribed to lower cholesterol levels are statins (e.g., atorvastatin, lovastatin, simvastatin), but they also have been associated, in some studies, with slowing the decline of cognitive functioning in people who have Alzheimer's disease. When taken for high cholesterol, statins help keep plaque from accumulating in the blood vessels. Scientists have also noted that statins appear to reduce the production of beta-amyloid and tau proteins in the brain.

For example, a study published in *Neurology* in August 2007 examined the brain tissue of people who had donated their brains after death. The researchers found that those who had used statins had significantly fewer plaques and tangles than patients who had not taken statins. Since that time, subsequent studies have not provided strong evidence that statins are an effective treatment for Alzheimer's disease. Like NSAIDs, more research on the use of statins in Alzheimer's disease is needed before we know if they can provide any significant benefits for these patients.

## DRUGS FOR TREATMENT OF BEHAVIORAL AND PSYCHIATRIC SYMPTOMS

Along with memory problems, people who have Alzheimer's disease also experience various behavioral and psychiatric symptoms. In the early stages of Alzheimer's disease, there are usually only a few behavioral and/or psychological problems, and they generally are mild. More serious and challenging symptoms typically develop during the moderate and severe stages of the disease.

Symptoms that develop during the early stage of Alzheimer's disease will likely grow more severe; thus it is helpful to find effective ways to manage them as soon as possible so a good quality of life can be maintained as long as possible. Management can include medications, which we discuss below, as well as complementary treatments, which are covered in the next chapter. Generally, it is best to begin with non-drug treatment approaches and turn to prescriptions if and when non-prescription methods do not work.

## DEPRESSION

The main psychiatric problem that occurs early in the course of Alzheimer's disease is depression. Depression is not only very common among people with Alzheimer's (it is believed to affect about 40 percent of patients), it also is frequently diagnosed *instead* of Alzheimer's, at least initially. A misdiagnosis or missed diagnosis of either condition is unfortunate because individuals do not receive the help they need.

It's easy to understand why people who have early Alzheimer's disease would feel depressed. Martin, a 71-year-old retired engineer, began to experience a noticeable decline in his memory around his 70th birthday. His wife, Clara, recommended they see a geriatrician, and after neurological testing, the childhood sweethearts were told Martin had early Alzheimer's disease.

Although Martin had been concerned about his memory loss before the diagnosis, he quickly became depressed after getting the news. "I want to be able to do the things that Clara and I enjoy so much," he said. "I'm still in good shape physically, but this problem with my memory is a crushing blow. It doesn't seem fair."

Clara tried to keep his spirits up by encouraging him to continue participating in their social activities, including weekly bridge games, ballroom dancing, and birding, but Martin resisted her attempts. Frustrated, Clara sought help from a psychiatrist, who recommended the antidepressant sertraline (Zoloft®). Martin didn't want to take the drug, but at his wife's insistence he gave in. After several weeks, Martin's mood improved enough that he was willing to return to his social life with some enthusiasm. Over the course of a year, the doctor needed to increase the dose slightly, and after nearly two years Martin is still taking sertraline and faring well with depression.

When doctors prescribe antidepressants to treat depression in people who have Alzheimer's disease, they need to be aware of side effects and drug interactions. Older adults metabolize drugs differently than their younger counterparts, and they also tend to be taking more than one drug for conditions other than Alzheimer's disease. Therefore, any and all drugs need to be coordinated by a physician to make sure patients are safe.

Antidepressants known as selective serotonin reuptake inhibitors (SSRIs) are commonly prescribed to treat depression in Alzheimer's disease. It isn't clear exactly how SSRIs affect depression. Scientists know that a neurotransmitter called serotonin is associated with depression and mood, and SSRIs seem to relieve symptoms of depression by blocking the reabsorption (reuptake) of serotonin by certain brain cells, which allows more serotonin to remain in the brain. More serotonin in the brain improves mood.

Along with sertraline, other SSRIs include fluoxetine (Prozac®), citalopram (Celexa®), excitalopram (Lexapro®), and paroxetine (Paxil®, Pexeva®). Although SSRIs can relieve depression, they are associated with side effects, nausea, dry mouth, headache, diarrhea, nervousness, rash, agitation, restlessness, weight gain, drowsiness, insomnia, and sexual dysfunction. As you can see, many of these potential side effects can worsen the behavior of people who have Alzheimer's disease, and so they should be used with caution.

Another type of antidepressants, tricyclics, have been around longer than the SSRIs, and they work differently in the brain than the newer antidepressants. Tricyclic antidepressants inhibit the reabsorption of three neurotransmitters associated with depression: serotonin, norepinephrine, and dopamine. They are associated with more side effects than SSRIs, and that is one of the main reasons they are not used as often in people who have Alzheimer's disease. However, because everyone is different, they can work better for some patients. The tricyclics include amitriptyline (Elavil®), desipramine (Norpramin®), doxepin (Sinequan®), imipramine (Tofranil®), nortriptyline (Pamelor®), and trimipramine (Surmontil®). In addition to the side effects seen with SSRIs, tricyclics can also cause blurry vision, urinary retention, disorientation or confusion, low blood pressure, weakness, and sensitivity to sunlight.

## Apathy
What's the difference between depression and apathy? People who are apathetic are listless and lack emotion, enthusiasm, motivation, and interest in their environment and/or people and activities. Depressed individuals usually are tearful, very sad, and feel hopeless. Some experts say that apathy is more common than depression among Alzheimer's patients. If you and your doctor believe it is necessary to treat this symptom, it typically responds to psychostimulant drugs, such as dextroamphetamine (Adderall®) and methylphenidate (Ritalin®).

## Sleep Disorders
People in the early stages of Alzheimer's disease often experience sleep disturbances, sometimes because they are depressed and/or agitated. Many patients respond well to non-drug approaches, which we discuss in chapter 6. If non-drug treatment is not effective, your doctor may prescribe an antidepressant sleep aid, such as trazodone (Desyrel®) or doxepin (Sinequan®). If agitation is also a

problem, antipsychotic drugs olanzapine (Zyprexa®) or quetiapine (Seroquel®) may be ordered. Other sedating drugs such as temazepam (Restoril®, zolpidem (Ambien®), and diazepam (Valium®) can cause memory problems and even agitation.

## CLINICAL TRIALS

Clinical trials are the best way for experts to learn whether promising new treatments and technologies are safe and effective in humans. At the time this book was being written, there were more than 90 drugs in clinical trials for Alzheimer's disease, and more were waiting for approval from the FDA to be tested in humans.

For research in Alzheimer's disease to keep moving forward, volunteers are always needed for clinical trials and studies. In mid-2009, at least 50,000 volunteers both with and without Alzheimer's disease were needed to participate in more than 175 clinical trials and studies on Alzheimer's.

### Types of Trials

There are basically two types of trials. There are treatment trials that evaluate existing approved drugs to determine whether they are useful for other purposes. For example, trials are being done to determine whether anti-inflammatory drugs that are used to treat arthritis might be helpful in Alzheimer's disease. The other type of trial is one that evaluates experimental drugs to see if they can improve cognitive function or reduce symptoms in people who have Alzheimer's disease, prevent the disease, or slow its progression.

Trials are also done in phases. Phase I trials involve a small number of volunteers and look at the action and safety of the drug in the body. Drugs that pass this phase go to Phase II and Phase III, both of which involve a larger number of volunteers over a longer period of time. These trials look at whether the treatment is safe and effective and what side effects it can cause. After a drug passes all three phases, the study team may submit its data to the FDA for its approval.

## Participating in a Trial

If your loved one with Alzheimer's disease is interested in a clinical trial, this is a general idea of what to expect. Study staff explain the trial in detail, including the potential risks and benefits, to potential participants and their families. Patients and their families can ask any questions they need to so they fully understand the study. Patients are asked to sign an informed consent form. Laws concerning informed consent differ among states and research institutions, but all are designed to ensure the patients are protected. If your loved one is unable to sign the form, his or her durable power of attorney can sign, although different states have different laws about this practice. Patients are then screened to see if they qualify for the study.

Although each trial is different, generally participants undergo a full physical examination and comprehensive cognitive evaluation. They are then given the test drug or treatment. Some patients may receive a placebo. As the study progresses, patients and family members must follow strict medication instructions and keep records of symptoms and any side effects. Typically participants must visit the clinic or research center on several occasions during the study for testing and to talk with the staff.

## Things to Consider Before Entering a Trial

Your physician can help you choose the best trial for your loved one. Some trials are only recruiting people who have early Alzheimer's while others are only interested in people who are in later stages of the disease. Some studies are localized and are only being conducted in one or several locations; others may have participating research institutions and clinics across the nation. Because there are usually many studies underway, it is not hard to find one that can suit your loved one's needs.

Clinical trials generally do not produce miracles. The test drug or treatment may offer some symptom relief, slow progression of the disease, or reduce the risk of death. The trial also may do nothing or cause some side effects. All of these possibilities are explained to potential participants before they enter a study, yet some people drop out of a trial when they realize they are not getting better. Some people are happy to participate because they realize that even if they experience only a small benefit, what scientists learn may help others in the future.

Trials for Alzheimer's disease are usually placebo-controlled and double-blind. This means that some of the participants will be given a placebo instead of the study drug, and no one—not even the staff—knows which patients are taking the drug and which are taking placebo. Not knowing whether your loved one is taking the drug or a placebo can be very frustrating for some people.

Many families say that the best thing about participating in a clinical trial is that they have an opportunity to meet and talk with experts in Alzheimer's disease on a regular basis. "I must admit that I really enjoyed the clinical trial," says Julia. "When I went with my older sister, who was diagnosed with early Alzheimer's six months ago, to learn about the trial, I was impressed by the people who were running it. We go back for evaluations every four weeks, and in between I can call and talk with the staff about anything that I observe or any questions. It makes me feel like we're doing something positive, even if it doesn't help my sister much in the long run. She's impressed with the staff, too, and so it lifts her spirits to know that she's at least trying something to fight this disease."

The Alzheimer's Disease Clinical Trials Database lists the trials on Alzheimer's disease and dementia currently underway at locations throughout the United States. The database is a joint project of the US Food and Drug Administration (FDA) and the National Institute on Aging (NIA) maintained by the NIA's Alzheimer's Disease Education and Referral (ADEAR) Center. If you and your loved one are interested in learning more about clinical trials and details about which ones are looking for volunteers, you can visit two websites: the National Institutes of Health at www.clinicaltrials.gov and the Alzheimer's Association at www.alz.org/alzheimers_disease_clinical_trials_index.asp.

## UP-AND-COMING MEDICATIONS

Scientists are constantly researching and developing new treatments for Alzheimer's disease, with an emphasis on those that can prevent or stop the disease in its earliest stages. Several treatment options are currently being investigated.

- Researchers at Mount Sinai School of Medicine, for example, reported in July 2009 that they had found a compound called NIC5-15 that seems to be effective in stabilizing cognitive function in people who have mild to moderate Alzheimer's disease. NIC5-15 is one member of a new class of natural compounds that appear to have the potential to ward off the formation of beta-amyloid and stop deterioration of cognitive functioning.

Although the findings are preliminary, the researchers are hopeful that further clinical studies will support them.

• An Alzheimer's vaccine was attempted and then abandoned in 2002 when four of the patients in the study developed brain inflammation. But new research is bringing hope to the development of a new antibody approach to Alzheimer's disease. In the July 21, 2009, issue of *Neurology,* scientists reported that subjects treated with intravenous immunoglobulin (IVIg)—a blood product that contains antibodies from donated blood—had a 42 percent reduced risk of developing Alzheimer's disease when compared with untreated subjects. The investigators looked at the records of approximately 85,000 people age 65 and older, 850 of whom had been treated with IVIg for various conditions such as immune deficiencies, leukemia, and anemia. They found that only 2.8 percent of IVIg-treated patients eventually developed Alzheimer's disease compared with 4.8 percent of those who were not treated with IVIg. This finding has prompted researchers to test the ability of IVIg to prevent Alzheimer's disease.

• Another antibody drug being investigated for treatment of mild to moderate Alzheimer's disease is bapineuzumab, which as of April 2009 was in Phase III clinical trials, the final step toward obtaining FDA approval. Approximately 4,000 patients are participating in this study, which is testing doses of 0.5 mg/kg and 1.0 mg/kg, or placebo, in patients with Alzheimer's disease who do and do not carry the APOE-4 allele. Bapineuzumab is believed to enhance the ability of the immune system to remove beta-amyloid from the brain.

- An antihistamine called Dimebon® (proposed generic name latrepirdine) is also in Phase III trials and looks promising for treatment of mild to moderate Alzheimer's disease. Study results published in July 2008 showed that Dimebon improved memory, thinking, behavior, and over-all functioning when compared with placebo. In fact, Dimebon-treated patients maintained the same level of function on all factors over 12 months of treatment. The most common side effect was dry mouth (18 percent of patients). The researchers also discovered an added bonus of Dimebon use: caregivers of Dimebon-treated patients saved about one hour daily assisting patients with daily activities when compared to caregivers of patients who received a placebo. Dimebon appears to protect brain cells from damage and enhance their survival by stabiliz-ing and improving function of the mitochondria (the energy-producing portion of cells). This drug action differs from that of currently available medications for Alzheimer's disease.

- Another experimental drug called tramiprosate has some potential as well. The results of a Phase III trial published in July 2009 noted that the drug reduced atrophy of the hippocampus in people who had mild to moderate Alzheimer's disease. This benefit was measured and identi-fied using longitudinal volumetric MRI (vMRI, which we discussed in chapter 3). However, the actual cognitive benefits are still uncertain, so the future of tramiprosate is uncertain.


## THE BOTTOM LINE

People who have early Alzheimer's disease have numerous medications at their disposal that can help slow progression of the disease and relieve associated symptoms. These medications can be used alone or along with complementary therapies discussed in the next chapter. These treatment possibilities can be discussed with your physician.

# CHAPTER 6

Treating Alzheimer's Disease Naturally

As scientists increasingly explore the potential virtues of various alternative and complementary treatments, they are uncovering the benefits of some exciting non-drug therapies for Alzheimer's disease that can improve quality of life. These alternatives include nutritional, hormonal, and herbal therapies, which we discuss in detail in this chapter.

Margie became interested in trying alternative treatments for her 81-year-old mother, Priscilla, who had been diagnosed with mild Alzheimer's about one year earlier. "Mom lives with me, and for the most part she's pretty independent," says Margie. "But when she started getting depressed and having trouble sleeping, I became concerned because although I wanted to get help for her, I didn't want her to take lots of medications, since she has a heart condition. I discussed my concerns with our doctor, and she suggested giving Mom the hormone melatonin, which helped regulate her sleep. Once Mom's sleep improved, her depression seemed to improve as well, so we didn't have to worry about treating the depression separately. I was really pleased that we didn't have to resort to sleeping pills."

It is important to note that many of the alternative and complementary therapies people use to treat Alzheimer's disease and its symptoms have undergone a limited amount of scientific research. Some of the claims about their effectiveness are based on testimonials and tradition. However, we present the latest information on these therapies and urge you to discuss them with your physician if any of them are of interest to you.

## HUPERZINE A

Huperzine A is an extract derived from Chinese club moss *(H. serrata)* and is a popular herbal remedy in traditional Chinese medicine. Scientists have discovered that huperzine A can inhibit acetylcholinersterase, an enzyme that breaks down acetylcholine. As you may recall, acetylcholine is an essential factor in maintaining memory and the ability to learn. Because people who have Alzheimer's typically have low levels of acetylcholine, taking supplements of huperzine A could help boost those levels.

An article published in the March 2009 issue of the *Annals of Pharmacotherapy* reported that preliminary data suggest that huperzine A may improve cognition in people who have Alzheimer's disease. In a review published by the *Cochrane Database of Systematic Reviews,* the investigators concluded that huperzine A appears to improve general cognitive function, behavioral problems, and the ability to function, all without any serious side effects.

This study supports the findings of a previous one, in which 50 people who had Alzheimer's disease were given either huperzine A or placebo for eight weeks. The investigators noted a significant improvement in memory, cognition, and behavior in 58 percent of the patients who had taken huperzine A. At this point, however, experts are urging that large, randomized studies be done to identify whether these and other benefits are truly possible with huperzine A.

## ESTROGEN THERAPY

The decline in estrogen levels experienced by women as they enter menopause and their postmenopausal years is associated with a negative impact on memory, concentration, mood, language skills, and attention. Research has shown that estrogen replacement can increase the levels of the neurotransmitters that are involved in memory, mood, and motor coordination, including acetylcholine, dopamine, noradrenaline, and serotonin.

There is controversy about estrogen replacement, however, because of the associated increased risk of stroke, certain cancers (e.g., ovarian, endometrial, breast), blood clots, and heart disease. These risks came to light following the release of the results of the Women's Health Initiative (WHI) in 2002. The estrogen used in the WHI, however, was synthetic, and this is where the trouble started. Some experts, including Gayatri Devi, M.D., an authority on Alzheimer's disease and author of *What Your Doctor May* Not *Tell You about Alzheimer's Disease,* note that the danger of estrogen replacement therapy is due to the use of *synthetic* estrogen (e.g., Premarin, Prempro), not bioidentical estrogen. Bioidentical estrogen, which is chemically identical to the estrogen produced by the body, is derived mainly from soybeans and yams and is transformed in the laboratory to mimic the natural hormone.

Because information about the safety and reliability of natural estrogen has not received much publicity, it is often up to consumers to ask their health-care providers about this option. If the possibility of estrogen therapy is something your doctor has mentioned or if you are interested in trying it, ask your physician about bioidentical estrogen.

Your doctor may also prescribe progesterone to balance the estrogen dose. In that case, natural micronized progesterone is recommended. *Micronized* means the hormones have been broken down into tiny particles, which makes it easier for the body to absorb and utilize them. Estrogen is also available in micronized form. Your doctor can write a prescription for natural hormones, and it can be fulfilled by a compounding pharmacy, which can make the formulation specifically for your needs.

## THE THREE BS: FOLIC ACID, $B_6$, AND $B_{12}$

This trio of B vitamins—folic acid, $B_6$, and $B_{12}$—all play a significant role in brain function and cognition, and so some health-care providers suggest that patients with Alzheimer's disease or memory problems should consider taking these supplements. Here's what some of the research shows.

Although there are no significant controlled trials that prove folic acid is important in preventing dementia and stroke, the experimental evidence is strong. For example, a deficiency of folic acid is associated with an increase in homocysteine levels, and an abnormal level of this cell-damaging amino acid is a risk factor for Alzheimer's disease (see chapter 2). Therefore, supplementation with folic acid may help prevent high homocysteine levels and thus Alzheimer's disease. Two other vitamins—vitamin $B_6$ and $B_{12}$—work with folic acid to bring down homocysteine levels. These three Bs may be helpful in warding off or slowing progression of memory loss and dementia.

A Dutch study showed that folic acid supplements helped healthy older adults preserve and even improve their cognitive skills. More than 800 people ages 50 to 75 took either 800 mcg of folic acid or a placebo daily for three years. At the end of the study, the people who had taken the folic acid had scores on their memory tests that were comparable to people 5.5 years younger. On tests of cognitive speed, they performed as well as people nearly two years younger.

Although the people in this study did not have Alzheimer's disease or other forms of dementia, the results indicate that folic acid is helpful in maintaining and enhancing cognitive functioning. Previous studies also show that people who have abnormally low levels of folic acid are at increased risk of experiencing a loss of cognitive functioning.

Dr. Devi suggests a daily dose of 1,000 mcg of folic acid, along with 50 mg of vitamin $B_6$ and 1,000 mcg of vitamin $B_{12}$ to help ward off high homocysteine levels. For people who have mild cognitive impairment along with high homocysteine levels, she also recommends a more aggressive approach—injections of $B_{12}$ and folic acid—until homocysteine levels decline.

## GINKGO BILOBA

Ginkgo biloba has a long tradition in Chinese medicine and in Europe as an herbal remedy for memory, depression, and anxiety. Within the past decade or so, it has been gaining acceptance in the United States for these very same conditions. The good news is, there are scientific studies to back up its popularity and the health claims.

Let's start with the most recent research, published in July 2009, in which investigators reviewed the results of

10 randomized, controlled, double-blind clinical trials of ginkgo biloba and dementia. The researchers found that overall, use of ginkgo biloba resulted in a delay in the progression of symptoms similar to that associated with the use of cholinesterase inhibitors. Since ginkgo biloba causes far fewer and milder side effects than the prescribed medications, ginkgo biloba may be a viable option for people who have early Alzheimer's disease.

The results of this latest study support those of many previous ones, including one conducted by the Alzheimer's Society and the Cochrane Collaboration and completed in 2002. In that study, the researchers evaluated 33 clinical trials of ginkgo and concluded that the herb can improve cognition and slow the deterioration associated with the disease, all without the risk of serious side effects.

The "secret" of ginkgo's ability to impact cognition has been credited to substances called flavonoids, plant-based nutrients that act as antioxidants. The flavonoids promote blood circulation in the brain, enhance communication between brain cells, help more oxygen reach the brain, and prevent the formation of blood clots. These qualities can help improve cognition, memory, and mood, and reduce confusion and anxiety in people who have early Alzheimer's disease.

Although there are many ginkgo biloba supplements on the market, the bioavailability of the standardized forms available in the United States can differ greatly from brand to brand. Look for products that are standardized at 24 percent to 32 percent flavonoids (you may also see them referred to as flavone glycosides or heterosides) and 6 percent to 12 percent terpenoids (also called triterpene lactones). These are the active ingredients in ginkgo biloba. Ginkgo is available in capsules, tablets, liquid extracts (tinctures, fluid extracts), and as dried leaves for teas. The typical dosage is 120 to 240 mg daily, taken in two to three divided doses.

Most people tolerate ginkgo biloba very well. Some minor side effects may include headache, nausea, and upset stomach. If you have a bleeding disorder or are taking drugs or supplements that can increase the risk of bleeding, you should talk to your health-care provider before taking ginkgo.

## MELATONIN

Melatonin is a hormone produced by the pineal gland, which is located deep in the center of the brain. The production and secretion of melatonin are stimulated by darkness and suppressed by light, which is why it is associated with circadian rhythm and the sleep/wake cycle. Levels of melatonin in the blood are highest prior to bedtime, and so it acts as a sleep aid by providing restful, deep sleep. When patients with Alzheimer's disease experience restlessness or insomnia, taking supplements of melatonin may be helpful.

Randy's wife, Milly, began experiencing bouts of insomnia about one year after being diagnosed with early Alzheimer's disease. Up until that time, Randy reported that his wife had not had problems with sleep, and that the insomnia had come on gradually.

"At first, she would be restless for an hour or so, and then drift off. But her inability to sleep just got worse and worse. Then she would be irritable and sleepy during the day, and she seemed depressed. When I told the doctor, she suggested the melatonin rather than a sleeping pill. I was glad she did, and just about a few days after Milly started taking melatonin, her sleep started to improve. Now she's sleeping through most of the night every night, and her mood during the day is better too."

Dosing of melatonin should be done under a doctor's supervision. It is usually given in doses between 3 and 9 mg per day, taken before bedtime, and tests show that it can be helpful as a sleep aid for up to three years. Melatonin is available in regular pills, time-release tablet or capsules, sublingual lozenges, and liquid. The time-release products may provide the most restful sleep.

Melatonin is usually very well tolerated. Fatigue or irregular sleep/wake cycles can occur if too high of a dose is taken. In rare cases it may cause confusion, vivid dreams, and nightmares, but these effects disappear after people stop taking the supplement.

## THE CAREGIVER-PATIENT RELATIONSHIP

You may wonder why we put a discussion about caregivers under "treating Alzheimer's naturally," and much of the reason has to do with a recent (July 2009) study in which researchers found that caregivers who have an especially close relationship with an Alzheimer's patient seem to have a positive impact on the decline of the disease. The study is believed to be the first to show that such an effect may occur due to the relationship between a caregiver and an Alzheimer's patient.

The researchers found that patients who felt especially close to their caregivers were able to retain more of their cognitive and functional abilities compared with patients who did not feel as close to their caregivers. The feeling of closeness was greater in relationships between a spouse and patient than between child and patient. In fact, the cognitive decline seen in patients who had a close spouse/ patient relationship was similar to that seen in patients who take FDA-approved drugs to treat Alzheimer's disease, including galantamine (Razadyne®), donepezil (Aricept®), and rivastigmine (Exelon®).

# TURMERIC/CURCUMIN

If you like curry, then you might be convinced to try curcumin, the active component in turmeric, which is the main ingredient in curry. Numerous studies show that curcumin may help the immune system to eliminate beta-amyloid from the brain and reduce the damage to brain cells caused by free radicals.

In animal studies, the scientists injected curcumin, and the compound was able to cross the blood-brain barrier. This is important, because it means that the herb can reach and impact the brain cells. Not all herbal remedies are capable of this. In the treated animals, the curcumin reduced the indicators of inflammation, oxidative damage, and memory deficits caused by beta-amyloid. For now, it is not certain whether curcumin can cross the blood-brain barrier in humans who take the herb orally. Such studies still need to be done.

Curcumin also works well when combined with vitamin D. In a study conducted at UCLA and the University of California, Riverside, researchers found that curcumin both alone and together with vitamin $D_3$ helped to boost the immune system to protect the brain against beta-amyloid. In this study, the investigators discovered that curcumin increased the binding of beta-amyloid to macrophages. Macrophages are "garbage" cells, because they move about and ingest foreign material, which helps remove them from the bloodstream. Vitamin D helped the clean-up process by stimulating the absorption of beta-amyloid by the macrophages in most patients.

If curcumin is an herb you want to consider, discuss the dosing with a knowledgeable practitioner. Typical doses are 1 to 3 grams daily of the dried powdered root, 400 to 600 mg taken three times daily of the standardized powder, 30 to 90 drops daily of the fluid extract, and 15 to 30 drops four times daily of the tincture. Both curcumin and turmeric are considered safe when they are taken at the recommended doses. Too much of either supplement can cause an upset stomach. If you have diabetes, you should let your doctor know before you take turmeric, as it can lower blood sugar levels and result in hypoglycemia (low blood sugar) when combined with diabetes medications.

## MAY BE HELPFUL, MAYBE NOT

In this section we talk about some alternative treatments that have been studied, some quite extensively, yet nothing definitive can yet be said about their usefulness when it comes to Alzheimer's disease. There are anecdotal reports from individuals who say they have been pleased when they have used these supplements, but hard scientific evidence is lacking. We simply present what is known thus far and let you take the information to your healthcare provider if you so choose.

### Vitamin E

For several years, doctors were told that vitamin E appeared to help delay the decline of functional activities in people who had moderately severe Alzheimer's disease, although there was no evidence that the vitamin helped slow memory loss or other cognitive problems. In recent years (2008, 2009) studies showed that vitamin E was not effective in the prevention or treatment of mild cognitive impairment or Alzheimer's disease. In fact, one study, published in May 2009 in the *Journal of Alzheimer's Disease,* indicated that vitamin E caused a greater decline in cognitive function than did placebo in some patients who had Alzheimer's disease. Until further studies are done that show different results, supplementation with vitamin E does not appear to be helpful in Alzheimer's disease.

## Omega-3 Fatty Acids

Omega-3 fatty acids are a type of polyunsaturated fatty acid that has been linked with a reduced risk of heart disease and stroke, and recently they have been linked to a potentially decreased risk of Alzheimer's disease. One reason for this potential benefit concerns one of the omega-3s, called docosahexaneoic acid (DHA; eicosapentaenoic acid [EPA] is the other main omega-3). DHA is the main omega-3 in the brain and it resides in the fatty membranes that surround the nerve cells, protecting them and their ability to communicate with each other.

It is well known that omega-3 fatty acids play a role in protecting against heart disease. In fact, the FDA allows supplements and foods to place the following qualified health claim on appropriate labels: "Supportive but not conclusive research shows that consumption of EPA and DHA omega-3 fatty acids may reduce the risk of coronary heart disease."

Thus the thought has been that since omega-3 fatty acids appear to reduce the risk of heart disease and stroke—and these conditions share many of the same risk factors as Alzheimer's disease—and DHA is so prominent in the brain, omega-3 supplements might help prevent or treat Alzheimer's disease.

The results of the studies of omega-3s and Alzheimer's are mixed. More than a dozen epidemiological studies have reported that abnormally low levels or intake of omega-3 fatty acids or fish are associated with an increased risk for age-related cognitive decline or dementia. The protection offered by DHA to nerve cells in the brain may be limited, according to some studies, in people who have the APOE-4 allele. Then in a review of 15 studies and trials published in March 2009, investigators found evidence that omega-3 fatty acids may slow cognitive decline in older adults who did not have dementia, but that they did not prevent or treat dementia or Alzheimer's disease once it was present.

For now, more research is needed to determine the role omega-3 fatty acids play in the prevention and/or treatment of cognitive decline and/or dementia.

## THE BOTTOM LINE

The use of herbal and nutritional supplements can be used alone or to complement medications used to treat Alzheimer's disease. In this chapter we looked at the alternative substances that hold the most promise, yet there are others under investigation and/or being touted as being helpful for Alzheimer's disease and other dementias. Among them are acetyl-L-carnitine, bacopa, choline and lecithin, DHEA (dehydroepiandrosterone), and phosphatidylserine. You may see more about these natural alternatives in the future, but for now, the evidence appears too weak to suggest trying them.

# PART III

## Living Well with Early Alzheimer's

# CHAPTER 7

How Loving Support Can Help with
Behavior and Emotional Changes

Dealing with changes can be a challenge, and when the circumstances surrounding those changes concern Alzheimer's disease and they seem to be out of your control, emotions can run high. Fear, anger, frustration, anxiety, and feelings of "why me?" are common. If you or your loved one is experiencing any of these or similar emotions, you are not alone.

Memory loss is one of the most frustrating things that can happen to someone. "Suddenly I feel like I can't communicate with people anymore," says Lydia, a 71-year-old retired florist who was diagnosed with early Alzheimer's about one year ago. "I used to love talking with the customers who came into the floral shop every day. I remembered all their names, and I could remember what their favorite flowers were and even their birthdays and anniversaries. Now when I meet some of these people on the street or in a store, I can't put a name to the face. It's so embarrassing and frustrating. I don't even want to go out anymore. And I know it's only going to get worse. I hate what's happening to me."

Lydia is experiencing feelings shared by millions of Alzheimer's patients and their loved ones. The emotional and behavioral changes that occur during early Alzheimer's disease can be challenging, but if they are met with understanding, love, and compassion, they can be managed. Therefore in this chapter we explore these changes through the eyes of people who are living with them and share with you how they cope, adapt, and even fight against the new directions their lives take as memory fades.

## FACING THE CHANGES AND CHALLENGES

The early or initial phase of Alzheimer's disease is an especially emotionally charged time. Individuals who have been diagnosed with the disease and the people closest to them, whether they are their spouses, siblings, children, parents, other family members, or friends, have embarked on a journey that is full of new challenges and uncertainties. The one sure thing about the times ahead—that the disease will progress—can make the situation seem hopeless. We want to show you that the time ahead can be fulfilling and loving. Yes, your quality of life and that of your loved ones will change. The tendency is for people to want to maintain the status quo—to stop time, keep things as they are. Although you cannot stop or control the disease, you can have some control over how you and your loved ones deal with it and the quality of the time you have together.

Gloria, whose husband Jerry has early Alzheimer's, put it this way: "Some days it feels like we take two steps forward and one step back; other times we just move backward, and then there are the times when we don't seem to move at all. It's almost like a dance. That's how I look at it.

"The important thing, I think, is that we have this precious time together, and we are doing everything we can to make the most of it. Jerry is taking memantine and ginkgo biloba and exercising every day. We do brain puzzles all the time together. We've been at it for just over two years, and I see a definite decline, but we're holding on and doing our dance."

Every person accepts, adapts, and moves through the early stage of Alzheimer's in his or her own way. Studies show that people who have been diagnosed with mild Alzheimer's usually stay in this phase for two years. Some people, however, are able to maintain fairly good cognitive function for a longer time.

The disease can also be deceptive: as Gloria says, "There are the times when we don't seem to move at all." These are times when people can be lulled into thinking that they have stopped, even reversed the course of the disease. Unfortunately, at least for now, no one knows how to make this happen. So you and your loved ones must learn to travel a rocky road.

What may you find along that road? According to *Caring for People with Alzheimer's Disease: A Manual for Facility Staff,* people in the early stages of the disease typically have the following behaviors and emotions:

- No desire to start anything new

- No zest for life

- Loss of judgment about money

- Difficulty learning new things

- Difficulty finding words and may substitute or make up words that sound similar to or have a meaning similar to the forgotten word

- Periods of silence because they are afraid they will make a mistake

- Short attention span

- Less motivation to stay with an activity

- Forgetful about where they have put items and/or they put them in unusual places, such as food in the washing machine

- Difficulty with logic and organization

- Resistance to change or new things

- Tendency to repeat questions or comments again and again

- Irritability, insensitivity, anger, and/or frustration more than in the past

- Difficulty doing routine activities and chores

- Hoarding items of no value

These and other behaviors and emotions are part of the journey you and your loved ones are on. Here are some ways to help you manage them.

## MEMORY LOSS

Memory loss and problems with concentration and attention are typically the first noticeable indicators of Alzheimer's disease, and people typically react to them with a variety of feelings and behaviors. One common reaction, for example, is for individuals to try to cover up their memory lapses and mistakes, hoping no one will notice and that their difficulties will go away with time.

George is a good example. The 73-year-old former U.S. history college professor noticed he was gradually having more and more trouble remembering names and dates, something he had always been a master at. He bought a day planner and began at first to put in social events, doctors' appointments, and important family dates, but after a few months he started to forget to write these things down. When he did take notes, he was repeating the same thing on several different pieces of paper, and then he would forget where he put them.

George also noticed that when he drove to the store, he had trouble remembering where he parked or what he needed to buy. Because he didn't want his wife Betsy to know he was having problems, he would tell her that he had lost his list or that the store didn't have what they wanted.

But Betsy had noticed the changes in her husband's memory, and at first she didn't say anything to him. "The truth is, I was praying the memory problems were just a temporary thing," she said. "I thought that perhaps he was a bit depressed about losing one of his closest friends and that his arthritis was preventing him from playing tennis as much as he would like. But deep down I guess I knew something else was wrong."

After a few months of finding notes in his clothes pockets in the laundry and others scattered throughout the house and office, Betsy gently but firmly convinced her husband to see a doctor. After George was diagnosed with Alzheimer's disease, he and Betsy decided that they would work together to make George's memory loss as manageable as possible. For Betsy, that meant one thing: working together.

"George and I have always been a team," she said. "I hate what this disease is doing to him and to us, and what it will do in the future. George always had such a sharp memory for dates and facts. Now he forgets family birthdays and we decided it was too dangerous to let him drive any longer because he can't always remember where he is or where he is going. Two things we have done are set up a large calendar in the hallway and post daily reminders on our computer to let us know what needs to be done each day. We have installed a computer program of brain exercises that both George and I are doing. I figure I have to keep my memory as sharp as I can. I told George, we're going to keep working at remembering things until we forget to do it!"

Memory loss can trigger many other emotions, including fear, anxiety, frustration, depression, and even hopelessness. Making a commitment to maintain memory and cognitive abilities as long as possible is one way to cope with these feelings. The brain exercises described in chapter 9 are a good place to start.

Seeking and getting support from partners, family members, and other loved ones is also recommended, but because coping with and managing Alzheimer's is highly stressful, seeking help from outside sources can be tremendously beneficial. Physical, emotional, mental, and spiritual support can come in many forms.

## DEALING WITH PERSONALITY CHANGES

"Joan always used to be so logical and reasonable," says her husband, Burt. "We've been married forty-one years, and we used to have wonderful conversations about world affairs, politics, philosophy, and just everyday events. Throughout our marriage we rarely raised our voices to each other. We respected each other, even when we disagreed. Now our conversations are strained and even combative. I can't reason with Joan anymore. I am having trouble accepting that she isn't able to make decisions or reason like she used to. I want so desperately to have a normal conversation with my wife, but it just seems impossible anymore."

Early in Alzheimer's disease, memory loss is typically accompanied by a decline in appropriate judgment, reason, decision-making ability, and sensitivity. For some people the deterioration of these qualities is slight and remains so for many months, even years; for others it is more pronounced and can place a significant strain on the relationship between the person who has Alzheimer's disease and others. For Burt and others who are faced with these challenges, accepting that the people they love no longer have control over many of their thought processes can be a very difficult thing to do.

The same difficulties arise when partners and loved ones of Alzheimer's patients are faced with personality changes. Alzheimer's disease can rob people of their positive traits and leave behind negative ones, such as moodiness, aggression, impatience, and rudeness. People who were once gentle-mannered and cheerful may seem to have traded in their personalities for someone else's.

Abigail felt like she was living with a stranger when her husband of 51 years, Edward, became very moody and impatient. "Ed had always been a patient man," says Abigail. "When his memory began to fail and he was diagnosed with Alzheimer's, at first he seemed depressed but quiet. We were both scared—and we both still are—but at the suggestion of our doctor we talked with a counselor a few times to help us better understand what the future held. We also started Ed on a treatment program of memantine and several vitamin supplements and decided we would try to take one day at a time.

"But after a few weeks, Ed began to change. Now he snaps at nearly everything I say and he won't let me finish a sentence. He alternates between being rude and impatient with me and being silent. Our kids don't even want to come over anymore because their father is so rude to them. We know he's scared and that he can't help it, but it's so hard to see the man I love turn into someone I don't even know anymore. What happened to my gentle, sweet husband?"

Fortunately Abigail had already made a connection with a counselor, and she continues to talk to her to help work out her feelings of frustration and anger. Abigail's two children live within a few hundred miles, and they offer their mother moral support by phone on nearly a daily basis. At the suggestion of her counselor, Abigail has also been going to a support group for Alzheimer's caregivers, and she says she expects to continue going "because the love and advice everyone shares helps me get through the hard times."

## CHANGES IN PHYSICAL INTIMACY

A very sensitive and highly personal issue for many people who have Alzheimer's disease is the decline and eventual loss of physical intimacy in their relationship with their spouse or loved one. Physical intimacy includes many things, such as holding hands, hugging, caressing, fondling, sexual intercourse, and even just being physically near another person in a loving or caring way. All of these expressions of intimacy can be compromised and change in Alzheimer's disease, even in the early stages, as the brain cells are damaged and deteriorate.

For some Alzheimer's patients, the need for sex or physical intimacy declines, for others it increases. In the early stages of Alzheimer's, patients are less likely to express their sexual needs in inappropriate places or ways, such as touching or hugging a complete stranger. If a patient's lack of sexual energy appears to be reduced because of depression, which is common in early Alzheimer's disease, then a couple may choose to try medication to see if sexual interest returns.

For couples who have had a loving sexual relationship, the changes in intimacy can be especially hard to accept. These changes can take various forms and stir up many different feelings.

### Stanley and Lyla's Story

Stanley explained how he was still very attracted to his wife, Lyla, and longed to be sexually intimate with her. "We were always very loving, and my desire for her has not faded. But over the past six months, Lyla has become increasingly distant. When I try to caress her arm or her hand, she pulls away. She doesn't look angry, but she does seem confused. When I try to reassure her, tell her that I just want to hug her, she looks uncertain, so I don't go any further. I really miss the physical contact. I feel like my holding her could comfort her and me, but she doesn't seem to understand. So I've stopped trying, and it makes me incredibly sad."

In Stanley and Lyla's case, Stanley discussed his concerns with a therapist, and they decided that Lyla's reluctance to engage in physical intimacy was not related to depression. Rather than resort to medications, then, Stanley tried a different approach. He knew that Lyla had an interest in art and that she had dabbled in watercolors at one point. So he bought Lyla art supplies and encouraged her to paint. The act of painting seemed to reduce her confusion and anxiety, and now Stanley finds he can sometimes put his arm around his wife without her pulling away.

"She isn't consistent," he says, "but most of the time she is receptive to my touch. That's such a big improvement. Even though she has become increasingly quiet lately and is finding it harder to complete her thoughts, she seems to find some comfort in my arms. I'm thankful for that."

We want to point out that research shows, as we explained in chapter 2, that a close relationship between the person with Alzheimer's disease and his or her caregiver, especially when that caregiver is a spouse, appears to help patients retain their memory and brain function better over time than those who don't have such a relationship. Therefore even when couples are not able to maintain the type of physical intimacy they had in the past, the fact that they have that history and that they can retain at least some of their closeness can be beneficial.

## DEALING WITH ISOLATION

At a time when people with Alzheimer's and their loved ones most need the support and understanding of others, that's when family members and friends may stay away. Alzheimer's disease frightens some people, and when people are afraid of something they tend to avoid it and isolate themselves from it. This does not mean relatives and longtime friends don't care; what it often means is that they are uncomfortable, they don't know what to say or how to act around people who have Alzheimer's. They may also be afraid they will be asked to "help," and even though they may have made an offer to help at some point, they are afraid they will be asked to do something and won't know how to say no.

Doris ran into this problem when she asked her best friend, Jeanette, if she could stay with her husband for an hour or so while she went to a dentist appointment. "Jeanette has known my husband and me for about twenty years," says Doris. "She and her husband Larry used to go out with Paul and me before Paul got ill. So when I asked her to stay with Paul for a while since he has now started to be afraid to be alone, I was surprised when she looked panicked and said she had to check her calendar. Then she said she had to go and that she would call me. That is so unlike Jeanette to act that way, and I realized later that she was uncomfortable about staying with Paul but didn't want to tell me. So I called her later and asked if both she and Larry would visit with Paul while I went to the dentist. I emphasized how much Paul and I valued their friendship and that Paul was still the same kind man he had always been, just that now he was frightened and confused. Both Jeanette and Larry did come over, and ever since then they've been more understanding about how I feel."

The isolation of Alzheimer's can come from two directions. One is when family and/or close friends withdraw from the Alzheimer's patient and his or her partner or caregiver. Alzheimer's disease has been called a family disease, because the chronic stress associated with caring for and watching a loved one slowly decline takes a tremendous toll on family members. In some cases, adult children withdraw from their ill parent because they cannot accept or reconcile with the fact that their mother or father has changed, and irreversibly so. Such withdrawal also isolates the Alzheimer's patient and his or her spouse, and no one wins.

At a time when the family or good friends should rally together and support each other, the relationships can become very strained. Good communication and a willingness to listen and understand can help prevent such a breakdown.

## Ned's Story

When Augusta's husband of 40 years, Ned, was first diagnosed with Alzheimer's, their son Tom, who lived within
an hour's drive, came to visit every weekend. Tom and Ned
both loved baseball, and at first the two men spent each
Saturday or Sunday watching a game or two on television, or they got tickets for the minor league games in the
city. This gave Augusta time for herself, but she was also
happy that Tom was keeping up his relationship with his
father.

When Ned began getting confused about the games
and got argumentative with his son, however, Tom suddenly stopped his weekend visits. "The first time Tom
called to say he wasn't coming, he said he had to help a
friend move all weekend. I accepted that. But then the
excuses kept coming, and I finally asked him what was
wrong. He said he was sorry, but that he just couldn't deal
with his father anymore, that he wasn't the same man he
used to be. Tom said he didn't know what to say to his
father anymore. I told him to just tell him that you love
him, or at least show him that you do by coming to see
him. Tom's wife, Pat, finally convinced him to visit once
a month, and she came with him each time. It wasn't
much, but at least he came. I really needed him more than
that, and I was hurt and felt isolated from my own son."

When feelings of isolation emerge, it is important to
seek help from outside the circle that has shut you out.
Once Augusta realized that she was not going to get
enough support from her son and daughter-in-law, and her
sister lived more than 2,000 miles away, she looked for
help from her church. She talked with her pastor and was
introduced to a group of church members who visited
with shut-ins in the community, giving caregivers some
respite. Augusta found a man in the group who loved
baseball, and soon he and Ned were watching games on

television once or twice a week, giving Augusta a few hours each time to go to a movie, shop, or volunteer at the soup kitchen.

"The funny thing is," says Augusta, "is that once Tom found out that his father was enjoying games with someone else, he started calling more often and even coming over more than once a month. I think he realized he was missing an opportunity that he would never have again."

Sometimes the isolation comes from the other direction: patients, caregivers, and/or loved ones distance themselves from others. They essentially create an island for themselves and keep other people away. This can happen when people are embarrassed about how the person with Alzheimer's disease acts or speaks. Frequently people who have early Alzheimer's stop going out socially because they realize their memory and ability to understand and speak are compromised. To avoid feeling foolish or uncomfortable, they simply choose to stay home and isolate themselves. Often they make this choice while living with their spouse or other caregiver, who then becomes isolated as well.

## Hilda's Story

Robert was at his wits' end. His wife, Hilda, had always been a social butterfly, helping with the kids' school activities, participating in book reading groups, and after she retired from real estate at age 66, getting involved with a dog rescue organization. Soon after Hilda's 68th birthday, Robert noticed that his wife frequently got confused when they were out driving, and that she was routinely forgetting appointments and lunch dates with her friends. She even missed some of her dog-walking sessions, which she so enjoyed.

"Hilda has always been such an outgoing, friendly person," says Robert. "She was a great real estate agent. But she was getting irritable a lot, not only with me but with store clerks and her friends. When I tried asking her what was wrong, she only got worse. One of her friends, Karen, had noticed the forgetfulness and irritability and suggested I take Hilda to a doctor. I was really scared because I knew that Karen's older sister had Alzheimer's, and although Karen didn't say it, I was sure she thought Hilda has it too. Well, I got Hilda to a doctor and Karen was right."

Soon after getting the diagnosis, Hilda said she didn't want to walk the dogs anymore, even though Robert offered to go with her. She also stopped accepting calls from her girlfriends and didn't want to go out driving with Robert.

"She basically cut herself off entirely from everyone except me," says Robert. "I became her sole companion. She wouldn't even talk to our son on the phone. In the beginning when her friends would call I would tell them that she wasn't feeling well or that she would get back to them later. But she never did."

Robert felt isolated and frustrated, and he didn't know where to turn for help. Fortunately, Karen said she would come over, even if Hilda didn't want her to, and just sit with her. This at least gave Robert some time to go out on his own several times a week. Karen and Robert were also able to convince Hilda to return to dog walking, telling her that her doctor wanted her to exercise more.

"The dog walking is something we do together," says Robert. "She does allow Karen to come over to the house, which helps me a lot, but she hasn't opened up to anyone else. I know she's scared and depressed, and so I try to understand that."

# WHERE IS IT? DEALING WITH HOARDING AND HIDING THINGS

Although Donna noticed that her mother had some memory problems, she didn't realize there was anything else amiss until a recent visit, during which she found her mother's shoes in the dishwasher and a shopping bag full of empty cans in the shower. "I immediately became alarmed," says Donna, "because I suddenly remembered reading something about how one of the signs of Alzheimer's was when people hoarded things or put things in strange places. I knew I needed to take my mother to a doctor."

Hiding things and hoarding can happen during the early phases of the disease and continue well into the later stages. These behaviors do not seem rational, but for people who have dementia, such activities have a meaning. Some experts propose that hoarding and hiding objects may be how Alzheimer's patients gather together things that have special meaning for them and somehow bring them comfort. Patients may also be afraid that if they don't take these items—even though their choice isn't logical to others—that they will lose them or someone will take them away from them. Hoarding is likely also related to the decline in brain function, as patients do not realize what they are doing.

Hoarding and hiding behaviors are often harmless, but they can be frustrating and disruptive for caregivers and loved ones. "My dad kept picking up anything that looked like a remote control and hiding it," says Murphy. "One day when I wasn't paying attention he had collected the TV remote, the two cordless phones, my cell phone, and my wife's mouse and hid them all. We couldn't find them, and we had to go to a neighbor's house to call my cell phone so we could hear it ring and find everything in the house. Now we have to hide everything from him! But because we now know where he likes to hide things, we got some old, broken remotes and phones and put them around the house. Now he collects them and hides them, and we take them back out and let him do it again and again. We don't know how to stop him, so this was our solution."

If your loved one is hoarding or hiding things, here are a few helpful tips:

- Lock up any money or valuables, such as jewelry, collectibles, or coins, to keep them away from the patient. Some people with dementia throw things away, regardless of how much they are worth, because they don't realize their value.

- Always check your wastebaskets before you get rid of the contents.

- Once you have discovered a hoarder's hiding place, check it regularly. Hoarders often keep using the same location.

- Check common hiding places, such as under cushions and beds, in cabinets and refrigerators, and in washing machines, dishwashers, and dryers.

- Get extras of important items that are easy to hide, such as car and house keys, eyeglasses, contact lenses, and hearing-aid batteries.

## PLEASE DON'T REPEAT THAT

"I expect my three-year-old granddaughter to keep asking the same questions over and over, but not my wife," says Gary. "Lately she keeps asking me 'Where are you going?' every time I leave the room. Sometimes I announce that I'm going to go into the kitchen or the garage and that I'll be right back. Then she'll ask me 'Why are you going away?' It drives me crazy."

Sylvia says her husband's behavior is driving her crazy. "Irving goes from room to room and rearranges everything on the tables and walls," she says. "He doesn't seem aware that he's doing it. When I ask him what he's doing, he just says, 'Oh, nothing,' and keeps on moving things. He has already broken a few things, which isn't a big deal, but I find it irritating. When he stops, he's fine. He still likes to read and we do jigsaw puzzles together. But when he gets anxious, and I never know when it's going to happen, he just starts moving everything."

A common characteristic of early Alzheimer's disease is repetitive speech or actions. Typically people with Alzheimer's disease keep asking questions because they are afraid or anxious. People in the early stages of Alzheimer's are generally aware that they are losing their memory and their ability to reason and interact with their world. Their world is gradually becoming a more frightening and alien place, and so they may keep repeating questions as a way to seek reassurance.

Repetitive movements or actions, such as constantly tapping one's fingers or pacing back and forth, can be very frustrating, as Sylvia discovered. One tactic that she eventually tried, and which can be very effective, is distraction. Whenever Irving begins to move the knick-knacks in the dining room, for example, Sylvia joins him and says, "As soon as you move that vase, let's go have some tea," or "Can you help me in the kitchen?"

If your loved one asks repetitive questions or is engaging in repetitive behaviors, here are some guidelines on how to handle these behaviors:

- Remain calm. If you get angry, your emotional response may cause the patient to get agitated.

- Do not tell the person that he or she has already asked the question. Instead, distract them with an activity, such as taking a walk, having something to drink, or helping you with a chore.

- Answer a question with a question. If someone keeps asking you "When are we going to the store?" and you keep responding with "We're not going to the store," this response can cause frustration. Instead, you can ask "When do you want to go to the store?" Some patients seem satisfied to answer the caregiver's question and then forget to ask their question again.

- Distract repetitive behavior by offering an alternative behavior, as Sylvia did with her husband. Suggest that the patient help you with a task or give him or her something else to do.

- Try to keep the patient's daily routine as consistent as possible. This is reassuring and can reduce feelings of anxiety and fear.

- If your loved one tends to ask repeated questions, do not discuss plans with him or her ahead of time unless necessary. This can reduce his or her level of anxiety and the tendency to ask questions.

- Note if there is something in the patient's environment that may be triggering repetitive questions or actions. For example, a suitcase may

trigger anxiety and questions about going somewhere, or having lots of knick-knacks around the
house (as Sylvia does) may cause a patient to want
to move them. (The other action Sylvia could
have taken was to remove all the knick-knacks
from the house.)

## THE BOTTOM LINE

We cannot emphasize enough the importance of reaching
out to others and of trying different activities that can alleviate the challenges associated with behavioral and
emotional changes that occur in early Alzheimer's disease. Often these approaches are the best alternative to
medications in the early phases of the disease. A detailed
discussion of such activities is presented in chapters 8 and
9, and sources of outside help are explored in chapter 12.

# CHAPTER 8

How to Live Every Day to the Fullest

Would you like to experience pleasure, excitement, and peace every day of your life? Do you think these experiences are not possible because you or your loved one has Alzheimer's disease? This chapter is about how to grab onto positive and fulfilling opportunities and help make the most of every moment whether you are the individual who has Alzheimer's disease or a caregiver.

We are not being Pollyanna; we know that Alzheimer's disease presents challenges to your life every single day. But we are saying that it is possible, and indeed desirable, to find and implement ways to improve the quality of life of people who have Alzheimer's disease and their companions. That is what we propose here.

Negative feelings can cause or contribute to psychological and behavioral problems regardless of whether you or someone else has Alzheimer's disease. Injecting positive, stimulating activities and moments into your daily life can alleviate some of the stress, anxiety, and frustration that having Alzheimer's disease brings. When Alzheimer's patients and their caregivers and other significant people in their lives participate in these activities with them, the time together can be healing, even if only for a short time, for all involved.

Let's take a look at some of the activities that can significantly reduce the negative feelings of frustration, confusion, anger, and hopelessness that affect both people who have Alzheimer's and their caregivers. Yes, everyone can participate in these activities, even grandchildren in many cases.

## THE POWER OF ARTWORK

Art manifests in many forms—paintings, sculpture, music, dance, and other creative media. Here we talk specifically about artwork created by hand—drawing, watercolors, ceramics, sculpture, and the like. Music and dance are performance arts and are discussed separately.

The mental deterioration that occurs in Alzheimer's patients changes the way they feel and experience their environment. Much of their frustration and anxiety is associated with their reduced ability to express their feelings the way they used to. Artwork, both viewing it and creating it, gives Alzheimer's patients a way to express their emotions in new ways.

### Going to the Galleries

People who have Alzheimer's typically develop what clinicians call "the four A's"—aggression, agitation, apathy, and anxiety. These feelings and behaviors are usually not severe in the early stages of the disease, but this time is also an excellent occasion to introduce a fifth "A" into the picture: Art. For reasons not completely understood by researchers, exposing people with Alzheimer's to great works of art has the power to make the four A's fade. One explanation is that while something like a movie requires people to follow it from beginning to end, a piece of art is stable and always there. This allows them to study it and let their interaction with it evoke whatever memories that come up. Some doctors call this "emotional memory," which is feelings that people have had earlier in their lives that are related to people and events from the past.

Taking trips to art galleries can be both a pleasant way to spend time with your loved one and hopefully trigger emotional memory and pleasant feelings. The art gallery need not be large. In fact, a big facility may be too over-whelming for some Alzheimer's patients.

## Creating Art at Home

Creating works of art, whether it is done with water-colors, oil paints, clay, charcoals, ink, paper, or other media, has been shown to reduce stress and depression and improve a person's sense of well-being and self-esteem. Working with art materials also improves hand-eye coordination and stimulates neuronal activity in the brain, strengthening the gaps between nerve cells. Art therapists who work with Alzheimer's patients report that their clients are less stressed and depressed and more sociable than patients who don't participate in art activities.

About six months after Josephine was diagnosed with Alzheimer's disease, the 71-year-old widow moved in with her daughter when Stephanie noticed that her mother was having increasing difficulty with her memory. "I was so afraid she would turn on the stove and forget to turn it off," said Stephanie. "And I knew it was time for her not to be alone anymore."

But Josephine's once even temperament and pleasant personality changed as she became increasingly fright-ened and frustrated with her inability to communicate clearly and to concentrate on reading, which she loved to do. Stephanie wanted to find something for her mother to do that would be stress-free and fun. She decided to try drawing.

"My mother had dabbled with drawing in charcoal as a young woman, but she started having kids, and then she went to work, so she gave it up. I figured the old desire and know-how was probably still there, so I bought some drawing paper and charcoals and gave them to her."

Stephanie also gave her mother "assignments" so she would have something to focus on. "When I first gave the art supplies to Mom, she looked a bit anxious. When I explained that perhaps she would like to draw again, she said she didn't know what to draw. So I gave her assignments, asking her to draw the vase in the dining room, the roses in the garden, and the birdbath in the yard. She responded to that, and now her temperament has improved."

If you would like to introduce your loved one to opportunities to create works of art, here are some tips:

- If your loved one has done artwork in the past, see if he or she would like to return to that medium. If they seem uncertain or hesitant, a trip to an art gallery may stimulate them to want to try their hand at creating art again.

- Allow patients to use "adult" art materials. Crayons, felt markers, colored pencils, and construction paper are often associated with children's art. Some patients, however, may prefer these items, so do not dismiss them altogether. Initially offer watercolors, clay, charcoal, or pastels.

- Establish an area dedicated for your loved one to work on their creations. Providing an easel can be a nice touch, if appropriate.

- Safety is of utmost importance, so avoid sharp objects and toxic substances.

- Keep your comments about the artwork positive. It is not necessary for the patient to finish any project or to adhere to your idea of what is right. Blue people and upside-down trees are perfectly fine because they are how the individual wishes to express him- or herself.

- Some areas have creative programs for people with Alzheimer's and other forms of dementia. Contact the local chapter of the Alzheimer's Association or talk to a social worker or therapist at a local hospital about any programs your loved one might be able to participate in.

- If your loved one agrees, play soothing music in the background while they create. Music can stimulate the creative process.

## MUSIC AND DANCE: THE POWER TO MOVE US

Martha had been very depressed ever since she got the diagnosis of early Alzheimer's disease. Her husband, Arnie, says he "tried everything" to improve her mood. "My wife's memory is not so bad yet, and I really thought she would feel so much better if she would just try different things. I felt like she was giving up. I spoke with her doctor, who suggested antidepressants, but I didn't want to put her on drugs.

"Then a friend of ours suggested music. Martha used to sing in a women's community choir for a while, and we used to go to jazz concerts occasionally. So I started playing instrumental jazz music in the background at home, and I was surprised, but she really liked it. Then she started asking me to play certain songs. She has trouble remembering the names of the songs, so it's a guessing game a lot of the time. But she's much more animated now, and she talks more. I even convinced her to go to a jazz concert in the park last week."

According to Concetta M. Tomaino, director of the Institute for Music and Neurologic Function, "Music . . . can provide access not only to specific moods and memories, but also to the entire thought-structure and personality of the past." Many studies show that memory and music are a healing combination. One of the most recent studies is from the University of California, Davis, in which Petr Janata, associate professor of psychology, showed that memory, emotions, and music all activate the same region of the brain, an area called the medial prefrontal cortex, which is just behind the forehead.

Dr. Janata used imaging to map the brain activity of people while they listened to music. He found that as Alzheimer's progresses, this area of the brain remains intact longer than most other areas. Other studies have shown that music therapy can be a very effective way to manage behavioral and emotional problems that occur up to the late stages of the disease.

## Dancing to Remember

Dancing is one of the most powerful activities for people who have Alzheimer's because it can do three essential things: provide physical exercise, increase the level of brain chemicals that stimulate nerve cells to grow, and help some people recall forgotten memories when they dance to music they used to know. To this list we also want to add that dancing is fun, and we want to add some pleasure to your life.

In 2006, Dr. Joe Verghese, associate professor of

neurology at Albert Einstein College of Medicine of Yeshiva University in the Bronx, conducted a study and discovered that dancing helped to reduce the risk of dementia. Dancing may have this power, he theorized, because, in addition to improving blood flow, it requires that people follow the music, remember the dance steps, and improvise as needed.

Music and dance can enrich the lives of Alzheimer's patients and their caregivers. Here are a few tips to consider.

- Choose music that the patient enjoyed in the past. This will evoke memories and can stimulate conversation, reduce anxiety and restlessness, and make the patient feel comfortable and safe.

- Play soothing music in the background, as it can greatly reduce feelings of anxiety, restlessness, and frustration. Eliminate other background sounds, because they can be distracting and disruptive.

- Encourage the patient to sing along, and don't you be afraid to sing along, too. This does not need to be a planned activity; just bursting into song while music is playing can be a great stress reducer.

- Attend concerts and/or dance productions if the patient is willing to go. Choose small venues, perhaps even outdoor events, which can be less threatening.

- Consider taking a dance class. The level of the class you choose will depend on how well you and the patient already know how to dance and how able the patient is able to participate. Be cautious if there is a risk of falling.

Music and dance are wonderful diversions for people who have Alzheimer's, and many patients greatly improve their mood and disposition while they are engaged in these activities. Do not be disappointed, however, if they quickly revert back to their prior mood or habits once the activity is over. Also note if the patient seems to be frustrated or agitated by any musical or dancing activity. If so, stop doing it and find something else.

## GETTING YOUR HANDS DIRTY

There is something very relaxing and soothing about working with soil and plants and making things grow. When people with Alzheimer's work in a garden, plant seeds, pick weeds, replant flowers, and do other tasks with plants, they have an opportunity to create living beauty, and to take care of it themselves. These activities can help build self-esteem, reduce anxiety, allow for self-expression, improve hand-eye coordination, and provide physical exercise.

For the first year or so after Earl was diagnosed with Alzheimer's, his wife Corrine says that he was in pretty good spirits and stayed busy by walking with friends in the park, reading, and volunteering at the soup kitchen at their church. But as he entered the second year of the disease, he became depressed and quiet, and it was harder for him to read and understand what he was reading. He wasn't sleeping well, and the lack of sleep made him irritable during the day. Instead of reading he began following Corrine around the house, and it drove her crazy.

"I had to find something else for him to do," she says. "The volunteer work was only twice a week for a few hours. I knew how much Earl loved flowers, but since we live on the eighth floor of a condo, it didn't occur to me that we could start our own little garden on the patio. But that's what I decided to do."

Corrine bought several long planters and lots of smaller pots. She and Earl went through seed catalogs and picked out the flowers he wanted, and then they bought some varieties that were already grown so he could transplant them to his balcony garden. "He was delighted," says Corinne, "but it wasn't enough. He was restless, and he couldn't very well pace in his little balcony garden. So I needed to find a big garden for him."

The chance came by way of a community vegetable garden that Corrine heard about from a friend. Although Earl said he didn't want to do vegetables, the head of the project said they needed herbs. Would Earl and Corrine be in charge? "Well, Earl was excited about that," says Corrine. "We planted thyme, sage, rosemary, parsley, and basil. Now Earl has two gardens he can go to, and he's much happier, although I've noticed that he can't always remember the names of the plants anymore. But he's sleeping better, and so am I."

Your loved one's venture into horticulture need not be a big affair: a few potted plants on the patio, starting seeds in small containers on a window sill, or perhaps a small plot in the backyard. Container gardening is popular, and some people with Alzheimer's like the idea of growing their own vegetables like tomatoes and lettuce in pots. Container gardening can be easier for people who may have difficulty bending down or kneeling on the ground.

## PUPPY LOVE

"Nothing makes my mother smile like that dog does," says Isabel, as she watched Darlene lead the golden retriever, Daisy, around the yard. "Daisy is a therapy dog, and she belongs to my boss," explains Isabel. "He brings Daisy here twice a week, and my mother looks forward to those visits. She always asks me, 'Is Daisy coming?' and I assure her that she is. Sometimes I wish she could come here every day, because my mom becomes much less anxious and depressed when the dog has been here."

Pet therapy is a proven way to brighten the lives of Alzheimer's patients. Many studies show that the presence of pets, whether it's a poodle, a calico, or even a rabbit or bird, can improve both physical and emotional health. Research has documented that blood pressure, heart rate, and respiration rate all decline when pets are around. Patients experience less anxiety and depression, feel less lonely, and have a chance to experience the unconditional love that pets can bring.

During the early stages of Alzheimer's, patients typically are able to interact with the animals more than patients can in later phases of the disease. Therefore, having a dog around can encourage a patient to walk or get other exercise by playing fetch or grooming the animal. Cats can be great lap and companion animals, and they may be better for a patient who is not as active. Ronald found that his brother, Steve, calmed down considerably when he bought a 20-gallon fish tank and stocked it with many multicolored fish and accessories. "Steve can sit for an hour and watch those fish," says Ronald. "At this point, they are better than any drug the doctor could have prescribed for my brother's restlessness and insomnia. Whenever Steve is anxious or can't sleep, he watches the fish, cleans the tank, feeds them, whatever. They are like a tranquilizer with fins."

After seeing how their loved one responds to a dog or other animal, some people consider getting a pet for their loved one. Before you do, match the animal's size, temperament, and energy level with that of the patient. Also consider whether you will be able or want to care for the pet once caretaking becomes more demanding or your loved one must go to a facility. Dogs can make great companions and provide a sense of security, and they require lots of care. Cats can be less demanding (no outdoor walks). Animals that are confined to a cage or tank, such as birds, gerbils, hamsters, and fish, may be best for people who are calmed by watching and interacting with these pets.

If having your own pet is not in the cards for you, contact a dog therapy group in your area to see if they can send a volunteer and his or her dog over for visits, as Isabel did for her mother. You can also contact the Alzheimer's Association in your area to see if they have a pet therapy program.

## FEELING FOR HEALING

Never underestimate the power of touch. Alzheimer's patients can feel alone, frightened, confused, and anxious, and sometimes just a gentle touch on the arm or shoulder lets them know that someone cares and that they are loved. Touch is a powerful healing tool, and sometimes we forget just how useful it can be.

Two specific touch therapies caregivers may want to try with their loved one are massage and therapeutic touch. Caregivers can learn the basics of both approaches in just a lesson or two, which certainly is not well enough to be an expert but good enough to share the touching therapies with the affected individual. Massage involves physically touching the patient, while therapeutic touch is actually a misnomer, because the practitioner does not actually touch the client/patient. Therapeutic touch is an energy therapy in which practitioners pass their hands very close to but not touching the body as they promote the flow of human energy. Thus a person with Alzheimer's who is not comfortable getting a massage may feel safer with therapeutic touch.

Evelyn suggested massage to her husband, Tony, who had been diagnosed with Alzheimer's three years earlier. Tony, a 77-year-old retired airline executive, was doing fairly well on memantine, ginkgo, and a vitamin regimen, plus daily brain teasers. Evelyn said her husband's cognitive decline had been "blessedly slow," although lately she had noticed he was increasingly anxious and was having trouble sleeping. "I thought massage might relieve some of his anxiety and help him sleep," says Evelyn. "Tony wasn't comfortable going to a massage therapist, however, so I went to a class at the senior center where they were teaching seniors how to do simple massage techniques. After just two sessions I tried it on Tony on his shoulders and back, and he liked it. Whenever he's having trouble falling asleep I do a little massage and he goes to sleep. Sometimes the touching makes him uncomfortable, so I don't do it. But most of the time it helps."

A few studies have been done on the benefits of therapeutic touch in Alzheimer's patients, and they show that the technique can reduce agitation behaviors. Besides the physical relief patients can get from massage and therapeutic touch, there is the emotional benefit. Touch therapies convey love and compassion without words. Both the giver and the receiver can share intimacy. It doesn't matter whether the touch is on the feet, hands, back, arms, or other body parts; the healing can occur.

The basics of massage, therapeutic touch, and another hands-on therapy, reflexology, can be learned from a book or video, but it is best to get instructions from a professional. You can check with massage schools (which sometimes give free or discounted lessons), senior centers, community programs, and local hospitals and clinics for help in learning massage, therapeutic touch, and reflexology. See the appendix for resources.

## YOGA FOR ALZHEIMER'S

You won't see study after study in the journals on how yoga can help people who have Alzheimer's. (There are a few studies, however, on its effectiveness for caregivers.) But if you visit some senior centers or nursing facilities or yoga studios, you may see this phenomenon in action.

Oftentimes there is lag time between when an alternative therapy or remedy catches on in the general population and when the scientific community gathers itself to conduct some studies to see if the positive reports from the "field" are for real. Such may be the case for yoga and Alzheimer's patients. Stories about yoga for dementia patients have appeared in the media from time to time, and the people who run the classes all say the same thing: many patients love yoga, it improves their mood and behavioral problems at least temporarily, and caregivers appreciate the results as well.

One yoga instructor who regularly sees the benefits of yoga for dementia patients is Patrice Flesch, a pioneer in this area. This Boston-based instructor has worked with Alzheimer's patients for nearly 10 years. The *Boston Globe* noted that "Flesch's holistic approach is unique. She treats her students in a way that lends them grace, dignity, and a sense of control over a disease that can often make them feel powerless."

Yoga can be an activity that people with Alzheimer's and their caregivers can share. If you want to try yoga, contact local yoga studios and community centers and ask if they have a program for people who have dementia or for seniors. You can also contact your local Alzheimer's

Association chapter and senior centers. Ask about the credentials of anyone who is teaching such classes and ask to sit in on a class so you can see the level of activity involved. Yoga sessions for seniors and people who have dementia typically are very basic, low-key, and relaxed, which is one reason why they are effective in improving mood, anxiety, restlessness, and sleep problems.

## SENSORY STIMULATION

Few things make people feel more alive than when their senses are being stimulated in a positive, exciting way. Exposing people to positive sensory stimulation not only helps improve mood, it can also reduce stress, evoke memories, and enhance quality of life. That's why we suggest you might want to create a positive sensory experience for the person who has Alzheimer's disease—and for yourself as well—a place where the patient and you can go to relax and to feel calm and safe. If you can, you might dedicate a room or area of the house for your sensory stimulation experience.

It doesn't need to be anything fancy or expensive; in fact, you can probably use things you already have around the house. If you don't have an entire room that you can dedicate to this project, you may be able to partition off part of a large room or the garage, or perhaps even set up the area outdoors.

You might begin by providing the patient's favorite chair or somewhere he or she can sit comfortably. Add items that make sounds that please the patient, such as music, wind chimes (which the patient can touch to create the sound), bongo drums, environmental sounds on DVD, or perhaps an instrument that the individual plays or used to play. Aromatherapy is a nice touch, and several essential oils have been identified as helping soothe patients and improve mood, including sweet orange, lavender, eucalyptus, and peppermint. These oils can be used in an electric or terra-cotta aromatherapy lamp or diffuser, or in a humidifier. (Because aromatherapy can help calm the nerves of everyone within sniffing distance, some people use aromatherapy throughout their home.)

Place lots of touchable items in the room: fuzzy pillows or stuffed animals, silk flowers, rug wall hangings, and velvet throws. Remember lava lamps? They can be very soothing to watch. Place lots of the patient's favorite pictures in the room on the walls and on tables and shelves. Put photo albums on the table so the patient can flip through them. For taste, how about a bowl of grapes or cherries, some sugarless hard candies, or some popcorn?

Not all people who have Alzheimer's are receptive to the idea of a sensory stimulation area. But those who are, and their caregivers, find they can be a handy refuge when the challenges of living with the disease every day gets them down. Your sensory stimulation area can also be a relaxing place for Alzheimer's patients to meet with other people in the home, because they may feel more comfortable there.

## THE BOTTOM LINE

We have introduced just a few of the many activities and non-drug approaches you can use to help an Alzheimer's patient and yourself live every day to the fullest. These activities generally can be easily incorporated into an individual's lifestyle, and they can provide many hours of pleasure for people who have early Alzheimer's disease. In the next chapter we explore activities specifically for the brain—brain exercises.

# CHAPTER 9

Exercise Your Brain

The results of study after study say the same thing: People who engage in activities that exercise their brain may prevent memory loss and/or delay rapid memory decline. One of the latest such studies, published in the August 2009 issue of *Neurology,* added further credence to this finding.

In the study, researchers monitored 488 people age 75 to 85 who did not have dementia at the start of the investigation. The individuals were followed for an average of five years, during which time 101 of the participants developed dementia. When six leisure activities (reading, writing, playing music, doing crossword puzzles, having group discussions, and playing board or card games) of the participants were evaluated, the researchers found that the people who participated in 11 activities per week delayed their mental decline by 1.29 years when compared with people who participated in only four.

This means, for example, that people who did a crossword puzzle every morning at breakfast, attended a book discussion group once a week, and enjoyed reading a novel three or four times a week were more likely to keep their memories longer than people who participated in only a few activities each week. The advantage of participating in such "brain exercises," said the researchers, did not depend on how much education a person had. The bottom line seems to be, "Use it or lose it."

Because exercising the brain is so important in helping retain and delay memory decline and, by extension, the progression of Alzheimer's disease, we dedicate an entire chapter to activities that can stimulate your brain cells. In addition to the activities in this chapter, there are many books that provide exercises and computer programs designed for strengthening memory and brain function. We have listed some of these resources in the appendix.

First, however, we take a brief look at a way to exercise your brain that does not fit into the "brain games" category: learning a new language.

## LEARN A SECOND LANGUAGE

According to Andrew Weil, M.D., author of *Healthy Aging* and founder and program director of the Arizona Center for Integrative Medicine at the University of Arizona, learning a foreign language can reduce the risks of developing memory loss, mild cognitive impairment, and diseases such as Alzheimer's. That's because the effort needed to learn a new language—which admittedly is a bit more difficult to do as people get older—strengthens the connections between the nerve cells (neurons) in the brain.

This process of strengthening the neural connections can help prevent memory loss and also slow the progression of memory loss or Alzheimer's disease in individuals who already are affected. And the good news is, you do not need to master a second language to benefit: According to Dr. Weil, just the mere act of attempting to learn a second language means you are "exercising more communication channels in the brain."

With that in mind, you may be interested in the brain game #4, "Translation, Please." You don't need any special second-language skills to do the exercise, but if you decide to try to learn a second language, this game can be a part of your learning experience.

## AN INTRODUCTION TO BRAIN GAMES

We have divided the brain games into three separate categories, each one of which addresses a different type of brain functioning that can be strengthened or stimulated: language, memory, and perceptual skills.

- Language skills are found in two main areas of the brain: the left frontal lobe, which houses the expressive part of language; and the left temporal lobe, which harbors the ability to understand language.

- Memory skills are stored in various areas of the brain. The ability to recognize faces is stored in the frontal lobes, while the language cortex is engaged when you remember a story. Touch is recalled in the parietal lobe, the ability to recognize an object lies mostly in the occipital lobe, and memory of smells is in the temporal lobe.

- Perceptual skills are those that you need to know to get dressed, find your way to a friend's house, and brush your teeth. The ability to perform these activities is found in the parietal and occipital lobes, and they work closely with the frontal lobe.

# HOW TO USE BRAIN GAMES

The latest research indicates that people should spend some time each day building their "brain muscle." These brain games are designed to be fun, and so we hope you will find that the time just flies by when you're playing them. Try to spend at least 15 to 20 minutes per day engaged in a brain game. Of course, you can play for a longer period of time as well.

Variety adds spice to life, and it also makes the neurons work harder, so we recommend that you choose one or two different exercises or games at each session during the week. Choose at least one exercise from each of the three categories each week.

Some of the exercises require paper and pencil. To help you keep track of which games you play each week, we suggest you write them down in a notebook. For games that require paper and pencil, we suggest you keep the copy of the games each time you play them. You can use a three-ring binder for this purpose. Divide the binder into three sections, one for each of the game categories, and keep your games in the notebook. This will allow your doctor to monitor your games.

Are you ready to play?

# LANGUAGE GAMES

## Brain Game #1: Counting Syllables

**What You Need:** Paper and pencil, a timer (watch, clock)

**What to Do:** On a piece of notebook paper, draw a line vertically down the middle of the page. At the top of the left hand side, write "Four-syllable words" and on the right side write "Five-syllable words." Then write down as many four- and five-syllable words that you can within a 15-minute period. Total up each list.

**Tips:** You can choose categories for your words. For example, you might list four- and five-syllable words that are animals, fruits and vegetables, or geographic locations. You might also choose famous last names or words you might find in a cookbook (e.g., oregano, thermometer).

**Things to Think About:** Play this game once each week. The next time you play this game, see how many words you can list. Do not refer back to your previous lists until you are done with your new list. Did you repeat many of the same words? Did you add new ones?

### Brain Game #2: Tell Me about It

**What You Need:** Someone to listen to your story; your dog will do!

**What To Do:** Pretend aliens have just landed in your backyard. They get off the spacecraft and immediately they are curious: They want you to explain every object they point to. They want to know what it is, how it works, what it is made of, who made it, who would use it, and what it tastes/smells/feels/sounds like. Your job is to answer all their questions in as much detail as possible, about one or two objects.

**Tips:** If you are having trouble getting started, look around the area you are in and pick an item to describe. Perhaps you can describe a sofa, vase, television, toaster, laptop, maple tree, or shoes.

**Things to Think About:** Play this game once a week. "Tell Me about It" helps people verbalize the thoughts that are in their head.

## Brain Game #3: Crossword Puzzles

**What You Need:** Crossword puzzles, pencil with a good eraser, crossword dictionary

**What to Do:** If you often do crossword puzzles, then go ahead and tackle ones at a difficulty level that is comfortable for you. If you are new to crosswords, start with less challenging puzzles and gradually increase the difficulty level. Using a crossword dictionary is not cheating; in fact, looking up words is a brain exercise, too. Crossword puzzles are found in most newspapers and some consumer magazines. Magazines dedicated to crossword puzzles and other word games are also available. If you are comfortable working with a computer, there are dozens of web sites that have crosswords you can do online.

**Tips:** Plan to spend about 30 minutes per session with a crossword puzzle. Do not be discouraged if you don't finish the puzzle; just come back to it next time.

**Things to Think About:** Do a crossword puzzle at least twice a week.

## Brain Game #4: Translation, Please

**What You Need:** a beginner's foreign language book (Spanish, Italian, and French are recommended); paper and pencil; a dictionary for the language you have chosen that gives both the language and English

**What to Do:** Find a word list in the foreign language book. Choose 10 words. If the English is given, cover it up with a piece of paper. Use the foreign language dictionary to look up each of the foreign words in the list and write down the translation. Then, write down 10 words in English and look up the foreign word for each one and write it down.

**Tips:** You do not need to have any foreign language experience to do this exercise. In fact, it is best if you do not know any foreign languages. We want to stretch your brain!

**Things to Think About:** Do this exercise once a week or once every two weeks.

### Brain Game #5: Scrambled Words

**What You Need:** Word scramble puzzles, pencil, notebook

**What To Do:** Word scramble puzzles can be found in most newspapers and on the Internet, and in puzzle magazines. They are usually grouped according to level of difficulty. If you have done word scrambles before, choose the level of difficulty with which you are most familiar. If these are new to you, start with the less challenging puzzles and advance if they are too easy. The beginner's word scrambles consist of four- and five-letter scrambles.

**Tips:** First try to unscramble the letters in your head. If you find this too difficult, write down the letters. Begin by doing five or six scrambles per session, and gradually increase to 15 to 20 per session. Here are a few to get you started. The answers are at the end of this entry.

1. oushe 2. seabn 3. tufir 4. pleam 5. astto 6. mafre
7. thirs 8. gnifer 9. liplwo 10. bwasuy

**Things to Think About:** Do word scrambles once or twice per week. You might time yourself and see how many four- and five-letter scrambles you can do in 20 minutes. Write down that number and see how you do the next session. You might also gradually add one or two longer word scrambles to each session.

**Here are the answers to the above scrambles:**

1. house 2. beans 3. fruit 4. maple 5. toast 6. frame
7. shirt 8. finger 9. pillow 10. subway

**Brain Game #6: Word Associations**

**What You Need:** Notebook, pencil

**What to Do:** In your notebook, make a list of eight to 10 nouns down the left side of the page. A noun can consist of two words, such as "kitchen table" or "yellow leaf." Leave two spaces between each word or phrase. Then list at least five words that are associated with each word or phrase. For example, if one of the nouns you choose is "bowl," some associated words might be cereal, round, glass, soup, and salad.

**Tips:** If you are having trouble thinking of nouns, these tips may stimulate your thought processes:

- List some of the items that are in the room or space you are in right now.

- Imagine you are in your favorite vacation spot. What do you see? Write down the nouns.

- Ask yourself, "What would I see at a ———?"
  Fill in the blank with words such as zoo, park,
  library, department store, baseball game, restaurant, beach, campsite.

- List 10 foods that are in your cabinets and refrigerator.

- List 10 items you would find in the grocery store.

**Things to Think about:** Play this game once a week. At
each session, add one or two more nouns to your list.


## MEMORY GAMES

Memory is stored in so many different parts of the
brain that we try and exercise as many areas as we can.
Generally it is best to do memory games at least three
to four times a week. Sometimes memory games can be
a bit frustrating, because your memory won't always
cooperate! That's okay, the whole idea is to stimulate
those neurons and try to strengthen the gaps between
them.

### Brain Game #7: Remembering Poetry

**What You Need:** A short poem, about eight to 12 lines

**What to Do:** Select a poem that has some special meaning for you; this will make it easier to memorize. If you
have never tried to memorize a poem before, the tips below may be helpful. It is recommended that you practice
the poem at least two or three times a week for about 15
to 20 minutes per session.

  If you need help finding a poem, there are many

excellent anthologies available in the library and even on the Internet. Here are couple of poems to get you started.

### The Deserted House
by Alfred Tennyson (first 3 stanzas)

*Life and Thought have gone away*
*Side by side,*
*Leaving door and windows wide:*
*Careless tenants they!*

*All within is dark as night:*
*In the windows is no light;*
*And no murmur at the door,*
*So frequent on its hinge before.*

*Close the door, the shutters close,*
*Or thro' the windows we shall see*
*The nakedness and vacancy*
*Of the dark deserted house.*

### The Garden of Love
by William Blake (first three stanzas)

*I laid me down upon a bank*
*Where Love lay sleeping;*
*I heard among the rushes dank*
*Weeping, weeping.*

*Then I went to the heath and the wild,*
*To the thistles and thorns of the waste;*
*And they told me how they were beguiled,*
*Driven out, and compelled to the chaste.*

*I went to the Garden of Love,*
*And saw what I never had seen;*
*A Chapel was built in the midst,*
*Where I used to play on the green.*

**Drink to Me**
by Ben Jonson (first stanza)

*Drink to me only with thine eyes,*
*And I will pledge with mine;*
*Or leave a kiss but in the cup*
*And I'll not look for wine.*
*The thirst that from the soul doth rise*
*Doth ask a drink divine;*
*But might I of Love's nectar sup,*
*I would not change for thine.*

**Tips:** Poems that rhyme are usually easier to memorize, as are ones that bring up fond memories. People memorize things in different ways. Some like to set a poem to music or a melody; others find that if they keep rewriting the lines they can remember them easier. Still other people say they visualize the words in their mind and remember them that way.

**Things to Think About:** The goal is to be able to recite a poem without having to refer back to the printed copy.

### Brain Game #8: Going Shopping

**What You Need:** You need to go to a grocery store for this game; also a notebook and pen or pencil once you get home

**What to Do:** Take a trip to a grocery store with your caregiver or friend and select one aisle for the game. When you walk down this aisle, focus on the different products and the brand names. When you get home, write down all the items that you can remember. If you only remember a type of product and not the brand name, that's okay. Just write down everything you can recall.

**Tips:** When you are in the grocery aisle, think about whether it contains a category of items, such as cereals, vegetables, fruit, etc. Also think about how the items are packaged: Are there cans, bottles, boxes, or a variety of packaging? Another tip is to note if you have ever tried any of the products in the aisle. This can increase your ability to remember.

**Things to Think About:** Compare the first list you made for aisle one with the list you make during your second trip to the store to look at the same aisle. Check to see what you remembered on the second list that you did not on the first, and vice versa. On subsequent trips to the grocery store, choose a different aisle and repeat the exercise: in other words, you will be making at least two lists for each aisle that you visit. You can return and work on the same aisle three or four times if you want to.

### Brain Game #9: Play Me a Melody

**What You Need:** Vocal music that you know and enjoy, notebook and pencil

**What to Do:** Choose a CD or album of a favorite singer and play the first few bars of a song. Turn off the song and then write down the words to the song. Do not worry if you can't remember all the words; just write down as much as you can. When you are done, play the entire song and listen to the words. Then play it one more time and sing along. Singing can help with memorization. Now write down as much of the song as you can remember.

**Tips:** Another way to play this game is to look at the titles of the songs on the album or CD cover. Choose one and write down the words to the song. Then play the song to see how much of the song you remembered. Play the song one more time and sing along this time.

**Things to Think About:** You may find that singing the songs, either out loud or in your head, is a great way to remember the words. One song per session is usually enough practice. Play this game once a week.

### Brain Game #10: Write Your Story

**What You Need:** A separate notebook from the one you are using for other games or a computer/laptop

**What to Do:** Write the story of your life, including as many details as you can remember. You may want to write about your school years, adolescence, memories of family events, jobs you held, friends, vacations, places you have lived, and so on. Some people say using a tape recorder helps them because it allows them to get out their thoughts without having to take the time to write them down.

**Tips:** Writing your life's story can seem overwhelming, but it is very manageable if you create an outline and break down the story into chapters or sections. There are several ways to write an autobiography. You can:

- Write about your entire life in sequence, from childhood to the present day.

- Begin your story at a later point in time and end whenever you wish. For example, you might want to tell about your college years and the first job you got after graduating. That may be as much as you wish to share.

- Highlight a specific theme. For example, if you were a teacher, you might begin by telling how you first thought about being a teacher when you were 12 years old, and then mainly discuss your life in terms of teaching: your college years, first years as a teacher, students you remember, places you taught, and so on.

- Write about the one person who most influenced your life and why, and then how that person's influence shaped your life's path.

- Choose a life-changing event in your life, describe it, and then write about how it changed your life from that point on.

Ask your family and friends questions about the past and what they remember about you when you were younger. It can also be helpful to look at photo albums to help stimulate memories.

**Things to Think About:** This brain game requires organizational skills, planning, and writing. Patients with Alzheimer's who write an autobiography create a gift for their family, a story that can be read by other family members and friends for years to come. Work on this project at least three days per week. This can be a fun family project that involves children and grandchildren. You may want to add pictures to your story as well.

### Brain Game #11: Reporting the News

**What You Need:** Notebook, pencil or pen, radio or television

**What to Do:** Listen to a news broadcast for five minutes. Once it is over, wait about five minutes, then write down all the main ideas that you can remember.

**Tips:** As you listen to the news, focus on any words or phrases that are especially interesting, different, or unique. These may better help you remember details about the stories.

**Things to Think About:** Do this exercise two to three times per week. Each time you play this game, you may find it is easier to focus on key words.

## PERCEPTUAL GAMES

The games in this section involve some artistic creativity, but you do not need to be an artist to do them. The important word here is "creativity," not "artistic," so have fun with them.

### Brain Game #12: The House That You Built

**What You Need:** drawing paper (plain paper larger than 8½" × 11" if possible), pencil, ruler, color pencils or pastels (if desired)

**What to Do:** Think about a house with which you are very familiar. It can be a house that you lived in (or live in now), or the home of a family member or friend. If you cannot think of a house that you know well, think about your first apartment or any apartment that you lived in. Draw the floor plan of the house or apartment. Put in all the doors and windows, appliances, furniture, and anything else that you remember. If you can remember the outdoor environment, add that as well: trees, shrubs, pool, fences, garden.

**Tips:** First draw the main outline of the house or apartment and add the rooms one at a time. This exercise can be done gradually over many sessions by doing one room each time. Be as detailed as you can. Close your eyes and visualize each room and the details. Perhaps you remember something special about a particular room or all of the rooms: a birthday party, watching television with friends, cooking outside, learning to cook in the kitchen.

**Things to Think About:** Do not worry about your drawing abilities. This game helps stir up memories, and it can be a good exercise to do if you are also writing your life's story, because it may help you remember some details.

### Brain Game #13: Jigsaw Puzzles

**What You Need:** A jigsaw puzzle (500 pieces is a manageable size), good lighting, a table on which to assemble the puzzle.

**What to Do:** Put up the table for the puzzle in an area that has access to good lighting (an adjustable floor lamp next to the table works best) and that is out of the way of traffic. Assembling a jigsaw puzzle is an activity that many people find they like to go back to several times a day. Working on a jigsaw puzzle can be addicting, so you should have no trouble spending 20 minutes a day putting the puzzle together.

**Tips:** Choose a picture that is pleasing and not too difficult, especially if this is the first time you have done a jigsaw puzzle. Begin by assembling the border and then choosing a section to fill in.

**Things to Think About:** Putting together a jigsaw puzzle not only stimulates the brain, it also has a calming effect. Completing a puzzle also gives people a sense of accomplishment.

**Brain Game #14: Recipes**

**What You Need:** Notebook, pen or pencil

**What to Do:** This game involves writing down the steps it takes to complete a task or perform an activity; a recipe for success, if you will. Everything we do in life involves a recipe: There are certain steps that need to be followed in a specific order if the task or activity is to be done correctly. To do this exercise, think of several common activities *(see below).* Then make a list of the steps you need to take to accomplish the task. For example, here are the steps for brushing your teeth.

1. Wet the toothbrush bristles with a little water.

2. Take the cap off the toothpaste tube.

3. Squeeze a small amount of toothpaste onto the brush.

4. Replace the toothpaste cap.

5. Brush the fronts of your upper and lower teeth with an up-and-down motion.

6. Spit.

7. Brush the tops of your teeth with a back-and-forth motion.

8. Spit.

9. Brush the backs of your teeth with a sideways motion.

10. Rinse the brush.

11. Put some water into a cup.

12. Rinse your mouth out with water and spit.

Some tasks will take fewer steps, some will take more. Begin with common activities. Here are some ideas for recipes you can try:

• Make a cheese sandwich

• Write a check to the phone company

• Make a cup of tea

• Feed a cat

- Change a light bulb

- Make a bowl of cereal and fruit

**Tips:** This exercise forces you to concentrate very carefully and think about each step necessary to perform a specific task. To make this exercise easier, try these tips:

- Close your eyes and picture the activity in your mind.

- As you visualize each step, open your eyes and write it down.

- When the list is done, review it carefully.

- Give the list to your caregiver or loved one. How did you do?

**Things to Think About:** Complete one recipe at each session, and do one session per week.

### Brain Game #15: Go to School

**What You Need:** This depends on the class you take.

**What to Do:** People who have early Alzheimer's disease are usually capable of learning new things. The best types of classes to explore are those that tap into the creative part of the brain or those that involve light physical exercise: watercolors, pottery, beading, quilting, knitting, scrapbooking, model making, woodworking, writing poetry, journaling, photography, and embroidery are just a few suggestions, along with tai chi, yoga, water aerobics, and ballroom dancing. If possible, the patient should sign up with a friend, family member, or his or her caregiver.

**Tips:** Get all the information about the class: when and where it meets, how many people are in the class, level of difficulty, the instructor's experience, and the refund policy. Ask about any materials that are required and their cost.

**Things to Think About:** Learning something new or brushing up on a talent can be very satisfying for people who have early Alzheimer's. Some people discover they have a talent for their new venture. It is important that should the patient become agitated, anxious, or otherwise uncomfortable once the lessons have started that you discuss the problem with the patient and, if the feelings persist, that he or she stop taking the class. Perhaps you can find another activity to take its place.

## THE BOTTOM LINE

People with Alzheimer's who do brain exercises on a daily basis have a much better chance of maintaining their mental functioning for a longer period of time as well as enjoy a better quality of life. These games can be fun as well as beneficial for the brain, especially when patients share them with their caregivers and loved ones.

# CHAPTER 10

## Plan Ahead: Financial and Legal Decisions

After you get a diagnosis of Alzheimer's disease, the last thing you want to think about is how you need to handle financial and legal matters, as well as plans for future medical care. One of the positive things about getting a diagnosis of early Alzheimer's disease is that it gives you time to have your, or your loved one's, wishes known and carried out. It is important for all concerned that the person with Alzheimer's disease share in the responsibility of making these plans while he or she is still mentally capable. This lets them know that their wishes and personal values will be respected, and it relieves caregivers of having to second-guess what those desires may be. It also allows caregivers to handle these complex issues before the patient reaches a more serious stage of the disease.

"It is very hard to do," says Natalie, a 71-year-old retired bookkeeper, "but I'm thankful my children and I have a chance to sit down and make plans while I can still help. It's important to me that they know exactly what I want when it becomes too hard to take care of me. Making these plans is bringing us closer together, too."

A full explanation of the financial, legal, and health-care issues that you will need to handle is beyond the scope of this book. We do, however, offer an overview of the options so you can start off in the right direction. You will need to consult legal and financial professionals to assist you.

## FINDING PROFESSIONAL HELP

Financial and legal professionals can help you manage the assets of the person who has Alzheimer's disease and help make long-term plans for health care. Today there is a growing number of attorneys, financial planners, accountants, and other related professionals who are familiar with or specialize in elder law, trusts, estate law, the complexities of Medicare and Medicaid, and other issues of concern to the elderly. Elder law focuses on guardianship, disability planning, and other legal issues that typically affect older adults.

You can find and choose these professionals much like you would select a physician. A word-of-mouth recommendation can be priceless here, and this is where talking with other caregivers and support group members can be very helpful. You can also contact the Alzheimer's Association, the Office of Aging, and other organizations listed in the appendix. Most states offer some type of low-cost financial and legal services as well.

When you contact potential financial and legal professionals, evaluate the attitude and helpfulness of the staff. Be sure to ask about their fees, whether you are charged for phone consultations, and what materials you will need to bring with you for your appointment.

To give you a heads-up, the information attorneys and financial planners usually need to see include details about income, bank accounts, loans, insurance policies, trusts, mortgages, pensions, and investments, and the patient's will, power of attorney, advance directives, birth certificate, any divorce papers, and a list of the spouse's assets.

Be prepared to take notes and ask questions during your appointments. When you and the patient go to the appointment, you may want to bring a family member or close friend along to help you, as it can be difficult to think of all the questions you will have under such stressful circumstances.

## LEGAL MATTERS

During the early stages of Alzheimer's disease, patients usually still have the ability to make decisions concerning their legal, financial, and medical needs. This is the time to make sure all the necessary legal documents are prepared and signed so the patient can ensure his or her needs and desires are known and met. These documents include a will, durable power of attorney, guardianship, living trust, living will, and health care power of attorney. We will look at each one separately.

### Will

If the person with Alzheimer's disease has not yet prepared a will, now is the time to do it while he or she is still mentally competent. Some people with early Alzheimer's have "good and bad days," and if this is the case, your lawyer may recommend that you have a psychiatrist examine your loved one at the time the will is executed. This is a precautionary measure if you think the will may be contested.

### Power of Attorney

There are two main types of power of attorney: nondurable and durable. A nondurable document grants a designated person the authority to act on the patient's behalf any time before the patient becomes incapacitated, but not beyond that point. Because Alzheimer's is a progressive disease, you will need to have a durable power of attorney drawn up.

A durable power of attorney grants the designated person (known as the agent or attorney in fact) the power to act and sign documents on behalf of the person who has Alzheimer's disease (who is known as the principal) after he or she is no longer mentally competent to do so. Any mentally competent person who is of legal age can have durable power of attorney.

## Guardianship

If for some reason the person with early Alzheimer's disease refuses to assign a power of attorney or is declared mentally incompetent, you must ask an attorney to petition the court for a guardianship (also called conservatorship). This requires a court hearing during which a judge will decide whether the patient is mentally capable of handling his or her own financial affairs. If the patient is deemed to be incompetent, a guardian or conservator is assigned by the court to care for the patient's property under the court's supervision.

## Living Trust

A living trust is a document that allows individuals (known as grantors) to retain control of their assets during and after their lifetime. The grantor names one or more persons, a bank, or both, as trustee(s).

The trustee(s) are required to follow the instructions named in the trust by the grantor. In some cases, the grantor asks that some of the assets be given to specific people while he or she is alive; in other cases, some or all of the assets are dispensed after the grantor's death.

"Setting up a living trust was very important to my father," says Nolen, whose father has early Alzheimer's. "He had worked very hard his entire life, and he wanted to be sure that his assets were distributed according to his wishes. I'm glad Dad was able to make his wishes known and set up legally."

## Living Will

Also known as an advance directive or health care directive, this document allows individuals to declare their wishes concerning health-care and life-sustaining efforts if they are declared mentally incompetent. This document is understandably a very difficult one for people to face. It is recommended that no one complete a living will without consulting trusted family members and/or friends, especially the individual who has been assigned medical power of attorney (see "Medical Power of Attorney"). It is possible that the person named as medical power of attorney may have to execute the living will for the patient in the future.

A living will outlines which life-prolonging treatments the declarant (the person with Alzheimer's) does or does not want applied when he or she becomes incapacitated. The document is used only when the declarant's ultimate recovery is hopeless, and typically two doctors must make this determination before the wishes stated in a living will can be followed. Because the requirements for a living will vary by state, it is usually best to have an attorney prepare it for you.

## Medical Power of Attorney

Also known as a health-care proxy, this document allows individuals (known as the principals) to name a spouse, adult child, or other adult to make health-care decisions for them should they become mentally incompetent. The person named as the medical power of attorney (known as the agent) should also be fully aware of the conditions stated in the patient's living will (see "Living Will"). This document does not give the agent any powers over financial or other matters, only health-care decisions.

A medical power of attorney gives agents a wide latitude concerning treatment of the patient. However, an agent cannot consent to committing the patient to a mental institution, convulsive treatment psychosurgery, or neglecting comfort care.

It is important to have a medical power of attorney because Medicaid regulations do not allow family members to make treatment decisions for people who are mentally incapacitated unless they have a valid medical power of attorney or a court guardian has been assigned.

## MONEY MATTERS

Planning for the future for an Alzheimer's patient involves having a good understanding of his or her current financial status and the costs of current and future care. Typically as the disease progresses, so does the cost of care. During early Alzheimer's, most patients live at home with a spouse or with an adult child. That is the time to explore your options for in-home care and nursing home care for when the disease progresses to the middle and late stages.

"It was hard for me to even think about putting my husband into a nursing home," says Patricia. "Right now Fred is doing well, and I hope that continues for a few years. But I know I have to be realistic. It's just that the thought of tackling the financial matters is so overwhelming to me."

For people like Patricia, it can be very important to

have someone they trust help them with their financial matters, in addition to a financial planner. This other person can be a family member, close friend, or an elder mediator (see "Elder Mediators").

## Elder Mediators

An elder mediator is an impartial third party who has been specially trained and licensed to help elders and their families handle issues common to senior care, such as end-of-life decisions, placement in nursing facilities, financial decisions, and medical preferences. Intervention by an elder mediator can be especially helpful when there are several family members involved in the decision-making processes and they do not agree. Since such discord is the last thing an Alzheimer's patient needs to experience, bringing in an elder mediator can be a wise decision for everyone involved.

Elder mediators typically follow a six-step process when dealing with a challenge. Here is an example of how these steps worked for Eileen (the patient) and her two daughters, Monica and Hady, who were having a difficult time planning future living arrangements for Eileen. At the time of the mediation, Eileen was living with Monica, and Hady lived only a few miles away. Eileen was still in the early stage of Alzheimer's, but her daughters wanted to make sure they had "plan B" set in place since they both worked full time and still had teenagers at home.

- **Step One**. The mediator explained to Eileen, Monica, and Hady how the mediation process would work and gave the ground rules: no name calling, no bringing up past hurts, one person speaks at a time, staying focused on the current situation, and speaking only for oneself.

- **Step Two**. Eileen, Monica, and Hady were each allowed to speak and present her side of the issue. Eileen said she never wanted to be placed in a nursing home; Monica felt very guilty about even suggesting that her mother would need to go to one someday; and Hady believed Monica and Eileen were being impractical since neither she nor her sister could quit work to care for their mother. After all three women stated their case, the mediator asked each one to repeat what the others had said so he was sure everyone understood how each of the others felt.

- **Step Three**. The mediator asked a few questions for clarification purposes, and then he asked each of the women what they thought might be some alternatives to putting Eileen in a nursing facility.

- **Step Four**. Hady raised the possibility of her mother going to an assisted living facility when it became necessary, while Monica questioned whether a live-in caregiver might be a solution for the daytime hours during the week and then they could care for Eileen on the weekends. Hady also mentioned that adult day care might be another option. The mediator waited until the women had offered their suggestions, and then he noted that there were community services available, such as Meals on Wheels, programs at local senior centers, volunteer centers, and church groups that might offer some assistance.

- **Step Five**. This was the negotiation phase, as Eileen, Monica, and Hady discussed each option individually and listed the pros and cons of each one.

- **Step Six**. All the women were able to agree on adult day care, Meals on Wheels, and contacting Eileen's church, which they discovered had a very active volunteer program that helped shut-ins. The mediator drew up a contract that outlined what the women had agreed to, and they all signed it.

## Defining the Patient's Current Financial Status

The Alzheimer's patient and the caregiver need to gather together certain documents and information to get an accurate picture of the patient's current financial condition. These items include but may not be limited to the following. These are the materials you will need to take with you to a financial adviser:

- All earned and unearned income: salary, pensions, Social Security, interest and dividends, alimony, rental income

- A list of current liabilities, including monthly living expenses (e.g., rent or mortgage, taxes, utilities, association fees, gas, food, medications, subscriptions), credit card balances, taxes, insurance, and any outstanding loans

- Subtract the total liabilities from the total income to get the amount of money remaining after all expenses are paid (the net monthly income figure)

- Add up all the assets, which may include real estate, bank and credit union accounts, stocks and bonds, health and life insurance, and certificates of deposit. The figure that you get, along with the net income figure, is the one you will need when applying for most financial assistance programs. In some cases, the income and assets of the spouse of the person with Alzheimer's is also counted.

## Determining Cost of Future Health Care

As the disease progresses, people with Alzheimer's need an increasing amount of care, and now is the time to calculate the anticipated costs of that care. Alzheimer's is both a predictable and unpredictable disease: predictable because it always progresses, and unpredictable because the rate of decline differs from person to person, and so the future costs of health care are difficult to determine. Some patients can avoid going to a nursing facility or stay in one for only a very short time; others require 24-hour care for years.

Lucy's family found a way to come up with a solution for their mother's future health care. Lucy had always been a very independent woman, and even at eighty-five she was still driving to the grocery store, going to church, and babysitting her great-grandchildren. One of her daughters, Joanne, said she began noticing that her mother had begun to call her great-grandchildren by the wrong names, and that she was putting items in the house in strange places. She and her brother, Charles, immediately took their mother to a doctor, and early Alzheimer's was diagnosed.

After the diagnosis, Joanne and her brother saw a steady decline in their mother's mental abilities. Because Lucy had lived in her current house her entire adult life, she had good friends and neighbors. Since she didn't want to leave the house, they decided to try and respect her wishes. After they reviewed their mother's and their own financial status, they made a plan whereby they and their four grown children would take turns staying with Lucy in her home on 24-hour shifts and hire a home-health aide when needed. Because they all lived within a reasonable commuting distance, they believed this would be a workable and affordable solution.

Lucy and her family were able to come up with a plan that worked for them, but every family and situation is different. Think about the following factors when you make your calculations.

- **Income.** What income will the person with Alzheimer's continue to receive? Does he or she have disability or retirement benefits? Will you or another family member need to leave your job to care for the patient?

- **Living arrangements.** What living arrangements will the patient need: assisted living, nursing home, living with a relative? Will the patient be able to stay in his or her own home and have caregivers live in? If the patient stays in his or her own home, what modifications will need to be made to the home to make it safe? If the patient moves into the home of a relative, what modifications will you need to make to that home to make it safe? Such modifications may include installing grab bars in the bathroom, adding a wheelchair ramp, installing an alarm, changing floor coverings (to avoid falls), installing safety locks on windows, the stove, cabinet doors, etc.

- **Medical needs.** Consider that you may need home nurses, prescriptions, a hospital bed, incontinence products, shower chair, wheelchair, physical or occupational therapy, and physician visits. Will insurance pay for any of these needs? If not, how will you pay for them?

- **In-home help and respite.** Will you need to hire home-health aides or a live-in helper? Will you need a housekeeper? Will your loved one go to adult day care? Will you need someone to prepare meals for the patient? What transportation options are available for the patient when he or she needs to go to the doctor or other outings?

- **Financial and legal help.** Will you need to hire a financial planner and/or attorney to help with financial and legal questions? Will you need help preparing the patient's taxes?

- **Nursing facility care.** Do you know the availability and costs of nursing home care in your area? Do you know what services they provide and which ones are extra?

## Paying for Medical Care

Both at-home and nursing facility care for people with Alzheimer's can be paid for either out of pocket, or through one of three types of medical insurance: Medicare, Medicaid, or private medical and major medical insurance. Many older adults have both Medicare and a private plan that pays for at least some of the charges not covered by Medicare. Given the fact that regulations vary from state to state and that health-care reform can always change coverage limits, it is important to consult with an expert who is aware of the current requirements and reimbursement procedures in your state. An attorney who specializes in elder law, a representative with the Alzheimer's Association, or your local Office of Aging may be able to help you with your questions.

## Medicare

To be eligible for Medicare, an individual must be 65 years or older and eligible for Social Security or Railroad Retirement benefits, or be a disabled person of any age. Medicare is limited in that it covers only acute rather than long-term or chronic conditions. For example, Medicare does not cover the cost of nursing home care, but if a person with Alzheimer's disease develops a urinary tract infection while in the nursing home, Medicare will cover the cost of treating the acute condition.

According to new Medicare policy changes that went into effect in 2002, Medicare beneficiaries cannot be denied coverage for mental health services, hospice care, or home health care solely because they have Alzheimer's disease. Before this policy change went into place, people with Alzheimer's were often automatically denied coverage for these services.

Medicare now covers "reasonable and necessary" services such as physical, occupational, or speech therapy; psychotherapy or behavioral therapy when administered by a mental health professional; skilled home-care services (such as skilled nursing or physical therapy); and doctors' visits. These changes were put into place because scientific research indicates that people with Alzheimer's can often stay in their homes longer if they have access to services that help improve their quality of life and activities of daily living.

Medicare does not, however, pay for prescription drugs for Alzheimer's disease, adult day care, room and board at assisted living facilities, or custodial care in a nursing

home, although it will pay for skilled care services provided at a nursing home or assisted living facility if they
are deemed to be medically necessary.

## Medicaid

Medicaid is a complex federal program and the largest
public payer for long-term care services in the United
States. It is the only major source of financial assistance
for long-term care for people who have Alzheimer's disease. Each state runs Medicaid under broad guidelines
from the federal government; therefore it is critical that
you check with the Medicaid requirements in your state.

If an individual meets the financial-need requirements
set by Medicaid in his or her state, the program may provide coverage for nursing home care, full-time home health
care, and adult day care. It may also cover inpatient and
outpatient hospitalization, laboratory and radiology services, most prescription and some nonprescription drugs,
transportation costs for medical necessity, physical ex-
aminations, and dental, hearing, and eye care.

Although the financial requirements for Medicaid vary
by state, here is a general idea of the program's rules:

• The applicant must have a monthly income that
  does not exceed $300 to $600

• The applicant's total assets (minus a primary re-
  sidence, one car, and personal possessions) cannot exceed approximately $2,000

Keep in mind that although Medicaid will pay for long-
term care, not all facilities and providers of long-term
care accept Medicaid for payment. In addition, many nursing homes reserve a specific number of rooms/beds solely
for Medicaid patients. Therefore, you may need to inves-

tigate several facilities if you are considering nursing home placement for your loved one. You also need to consider what your options are if you cannot find a facility that takes Medicaid or if you have to wait for such a facility to have an opening.

Because of the financial requirements for Medicaid, many people become eligible only after they have depleted their own financial resources and assets and are below the federal poverty level. If the Alzheimer's patient is married, the spouse's income and assets are taken into consideration when determining the patient's eligibility for Medicaid. This does not mean that a spouse must deplete their resources before the patient can become eligible for Medicaid, however. If the assets of patient, spouse, or both can be transferred to an adult child, for example, then they will not be counted in the calculations for the patient's eligibility for Medicaid.

There is a catch, however, though Louis and his daughters were able to beat it. As soon as Darla and Peggy's father, Louis, was diagnosed with early Alzheimer's, the 77-year-old widower announced that he wanted to meet with a financial adviser. "Dad was always a planner," says Darla. "He never liked to leave anything to chance. So he was no different when he discovered he had Alzheimer's." Louis transferred the majority of his assets to his two daughters' names, including his home. He moved into an apartment near Peggy because he insisted on taking care of himself as long as he could. More than five years after his diagnosis, Louis is just now reaching the point where he needs supervision, so he has moved in with Peggy for now.

If Louis ever needs to go on Medicaid, he knows that he protected his assets. How? Because he transferred them to his daughters more than five years ago, he met the requirement for avoiding having his assets included in the qualification process. This is a condition you should keep in mind. If you apply for Medicaid, the Medicaid officials will look for any transfer of cash or property you may have made from the Alzheimer's patient to third parties (including friends or family members) in the previous five years of the date of your application. If any transfers were made during that time, the application is disqualified for Medicaid eligibility. However, the patient can apply again when he or she meets the five-year limit. Thus if someone made a transfer in June 2005, they could apply for Medicaid and be eligible after June 2010. If an Alzheimer's patient needs financial assistance for medical costs and the five-year requirement has not yet been met, then he or she will need to have other resources to meet those costs.

That's why what Louis and his family did was so important: They planned ahead when Louis was in the early stages of Alzheimer's. If you think your loved one may need to apply for Medicaid someday and there are assets to consider, you may want to consult a financial planner, attorney, or other professional who is knowledgeable about Medicaid regulations to help you with those decisions.

## Medigap Insurance

Several other types of insurance may be used to pay for an Alzheimer's patient's care. Medigap is a "secondary" insurance that you can add to a person's Medicare coverage. It is sold by private health insurance brokers and available across the nation. Federal and state laws dictate what Medigap policies must cover, including the deductible associated with hospitalization and the coinsurance or remaining hospital costs that Medicare does not cover. Some Medigap plans offer more extensive coverage, including in-home services and assisted-living deductibles. It is important that you get a complete and detailed list of what is and what is not covered in any Medigap plan.

## Disability Insurance

Disability insurance can be helpful if the plan was acquired before the individual was diagnosed with Alzheimer's disease. Once a diagnosis has been given, most insurers will not accept a new applicant. Another option is the government's Social Security Disability Income. People with Alzheimer's who do not have disability insurance may quality for this program. You should talk with a representative of the Society Security program to get details about the benefits and requirements, as they differ greatly by individual.

## Long-term Care Insurance

"I thought we were completely covered," says Madelaine. "My husband had been paying on a long-term care insurance policy for years, so when we were evaluating our possible future medical costs, we believed this policy would cover the nursing home. Well, when we took a closer look we discovered we were wrong. Because we did not have an inflation rider on the policy, it would only pay out nursing home costs based on 1970 prices. And that wasn't going to help us much!"

If your loved one has a long-term care policy, read the terms carefully to determine if the costs for long-term nursing facility care will be covered adequately. If the Alzheimer's patient does not have long-term care insurance, it is virtually impossible to get coverage once a person has been diagnosed with the disease.

## THE BOTTOM LINE

It is a sign of respect and love to tackle the questions surrounding financial and legal issues while the person with Alzheimer's can be a part of the decision process, and wise because it will take away the pressure of having to deal with these complex matters once the Alzheimer's patient requires more significant care. Financial and legal matters can take many months to arrange properly, and getting an early start allows time for any hurdles to be cleared without too much stress on the patient and his or her family. Another area that should be addressed during this time is future health care and living arrangements, which we discuss in the next chapter.

# CHAPTER 11

Plan Ahead: Care and
Living Arrangements

Most caregivers reach a point where they need to find either part-time or permanent full-time care for the person who has Alzheimer's disease. Many caregivers are spouses, who often are elderly and may have health issues of their own that do not allow them to care adequately for their spouse beyond a certain point. Other caregivers, including children and friends, often work or have lifestyles that limit their ability to care full- or part-time for the Alzheimer's patient once the disease has progressed to a more serious stage.

Thinking about and making decisions concerning a change in living arrangements at some future time is never easy for Alzheimer's patients or for their caregivers and family. However, the best time to make these decisions is during the early stages of the disease, when the patient can have a say in the plans and everyone else knows that they have time to carefully and methodically look at the options instead of waiting until it becomes an urgent situation. Planning ahead is also important because many facilities have waiting lists and/or may have a limited number of rooms or beds dedicated to Medicaid patients.

There are a variety of options available to patients and their caregivers, and some of them can be used in combination. Below is an explanation of the options available.

## IN-HOME HELP

In-home assistance can allow the person with Alzheimer's to remain at home, whether it is his or her own home or the home of an adult child, for as long as possible. Depending on your finances and need, you can hire a homemaker to help with housekeeping tasks, such as laundry, cooking, and cleaning; a home-health aide who can assist with bathing, dressing, eating, and personal hygiene; or companions that can help with supervision and recreation. Some home-health agencies have workers who have been trained by local chapters of the Alzheimer's Association of the Alzheimer's Disease Education and Referral Center, so this is one of the questions you should ask when deciding on in-home help.

You may also need health-care professionals from time to time, including nurses, physicians, physical therapists, and social workers. Check to see if your insurance will pay for such visits and if not, make sure you know all the costs of such services.

If you decide to hire someone privately (not from an agency or health-care facility), you will be acting as an employer and thus responsible for following state and federal payroll requirements, including Social Security, and filing the appropriate forms with the government.

Before you hire any in-home help, consider the following points:

- If you use an agency, check it out with your state's licensing board to be sure they are licensed and accredited to provide home care.

- Ask about how much training the staff has and how they are trained.

- Make sure you have a clear idea of how much the agency charges and what may or may not be covered by insurance.

- Have a clear idea of the duties you want the person to perform. Make a list of these tasks and discuss them with the home-care worker so you both know what is expected.

- Keep an accurate record of the hours worked and check them against the agency's or worker's invoice.

- If possible, occasionally drop in on the health-care worker during his or her working hours, or have a friend do it for you.

## ADULT DAY CARE FACILITIES

Many communities have adult day care facilities, which can be either public or private, nonprofit or for-profit. There are three types of adult day care facilities: social, health, and a combination of the two. Most of these facilities operate during daytime hours, Monday through Friday, although there are exceptions. According to the National Adult Day Services Association, there are approximately 4,000 adult day care centers in the United States, and they have been growing in popularity.

"Adult day care has been a godsend for me," says Ethel. "My daughter and I looked at several day care facilities when my husband, Harold, was still in the early stages of Alzheimer's, because I wanted to see what they were like.

I visited the two in my area, and I was impressed with both. So when Harold became a little more difficult for me to handle, I signed him up for adult day health care. Now I have the days to myself and my daughter helps on weekends. For now, until Harold gets worse, this is a great arrangement."

To be a candidate for adult day care, individuals must be mobile with the possible assistance of a cane, walker, or wheelchair, and in most cases they must be continent. Although they can be both physically and cognitively challenged, they cannot require 24-hour supervision. Social adult day care centers offer recreational and social activities, while adult day health centers often provide physical, speech, and occupational therapy and a staff of nurses and other health professionals. Patients usually need to be assessed by a physician before being admitted to an adult day health center. A third type of day care center provides both social and health services specifically for people with Alzheimer's or other dementias. Not all communities have the third type of center, so you may need to investigate how appropriate other available centers may be for your needs.

When evaluating an adult day care center (social, health, or both), consider the following factors:

- **Hours of operation**. Ask about the hours of operation. If you work until six every evening, you need a facility that is open late, or you will need to make arrangements for your loved one to be transported to a safe place until you get back home.

- **Transportation**. Some facilities offer transportation to and from the patient's home. Ask whether this service is available, and if it is, is there an extra charge.

- **Level of care**. Each facility has a list of behaviors they will and will not accept. Talk to the administrator of the day care center about their list.

- **Costs**. Centers that are run by local, state, or county governments or by a university or non-profit typically charge a nominal fee, while privately owned centers may charge more. Some centers charge separately for meals while others include them. Make sure you understand the fee structure and what it includes.

- **Activities**. Make sure the center offers activities that your loved one enjoys. Peter's mother loves music, so choosing a center that has a musical activity every day is important for him. Mary was concerned that her father was not getting enough exercise, so she chose a center that held stretching and gentle aerobics every day. The big selling point for Cecilia was pet therapy: the center near her had an agency come in once a week with dogs and cats, and her mother loved this activity the best.

- **Caregivers**. A good adult day care center allows caregivers to come and participate in the activities with their loved ones, especially in the beginning until the patient becomes familiar and comfortable with the facility. Ask about the center's policy on this issue.

To find adult day care centers in your area, ask for recommendations from your health-care providers, social worker, people in your support group, or your local Alzheimer's Association chapter.

## LIFE-CARE FACILITIES

The concept behind life-care facilities is that people can move into the independent living portion of the campus and then move to assisted living if their health worsens, and then to the nursing facilities on the same campus as their health declines further. Not all life-care facilities offer the same level of nursing care, and some do not provide care for people with Alzheimer's. It is not necessary to begin your association with a life-care facility at the independent living stage, or even the assisted living stage, but those who are already living on campus usually have first choice for a vacancy when one opens up. If you are considering a life-care facility, examine the contract and policies carefully. You and your loved one should visit any facility you are considering and ask questions (see the questions under "Nursing Homes").

Life-care facilities usually require an initial down payment plus a monthly charge for their services. Additional fees may be required for nursing care. You should have an attorney review any papers from a life-care facility before you sign anything.

## NURSING HOMES

Making a decision about nursing home care is one of the most difficult things you may have to do. During the early stage of Alzheimer's, you do not want to believe that your loved one may someday need to live in a nursing facility. The truth is, not all Alzheimer's patients do. For people with Alzheimer's who reach the stage where they need continuous medical and nursing care and monitoring to ensure their safety, a skilled care facility is frequently the answer.

You may wonder why you should begin to consider nursing home care while your loved one is in the early stages of the disease. Similar to the case with life-care facilities, it can take months, sometimes years, to find the right facility, there are often waiting lists, and not all nursing facilities have an Alzheimer's unit.

Nursing homes generally fall into one of three categories: private for-profit, voluntary homes operated by communal or religious organizations, and nonprofits run by government agencies. Regardless of the type of nursing home, they all are required to meet both state and local standards.

There are two basic types of nursing care facilities that can care for Alzheimer's patients.

- *Skilled care* facilities are generally paid for by Medicare for approximately 100 days, so they are not suitable for long-term needs. These facilities, which are also known as "sub-acute" facilities, only offer care that can be provided by doctors, licensed nurses, physical or occupational therapists, respiratory therapists, or social workers.

- *Long-term care* facilities are designed for people who require 24-hour care to ensure their safety. Medicare does not cover care in a long-term Alzheimer's nursing home, so you must use your own resources to fund this level of care. Many long-term care facilities accept Medicaid patients, but the number of beds/rooms available

for Alzheimer's patients on Medicaid may be
limited.

In fact, nine out of 10 nursing homes that accept private-
pay patients also participate in the Medicaid program. If
your loved one is not on Medicaid when he or she moves
into one of these homes, they cannot be discharged later
if their finances run out and they need to go on Medicaid.
Some nursing homes, however, will move a resident, without asking permission from anyone, into a lower-cost room
or into a special Medicaid section of the facility.

To begin your search for a nursing facility, you can
begin by getting referrals from your physician, social
workers, and your local Alzheimer's Association. Many
people find, however, that the most useful information they
get on selecting a nursing facility comes from other caregivers, including people you may meet at support group
meetings. These individuals have "been in the trenches,"
so to speak, and can tell you about their personal experiences with a facility.

Once you have a list of a few facilities, contact the administrator at each one and ask about their fees and financial arrangements, how many beds they have available for
Alzheimer's patients, the level of care, and the length of
the waiting list. If the answers you get are satisfactory, set
up an appointment to tour each facility. Your loved one
may or may not want to go with you on these initial tours;
this is a decision you and the person with Alzheimer's
need to make together.

If after the initial tour of one or more facilities you find
any that you would seriously consider, you can make several more trips to those homes, but these visits should be
unannounced and at different times of the day (e.g., during
lunch, during activity periods) so you can get a real sense

of how the facility operates and how the employees interact with the residents.

Visiting nursing homes can be a very stressful task, so we recommend that you bring a trusted friend or family member with you as a second set of eyes and ears. Ruth says that she didn't think she could handle going into nursing homes alone, so she recruited her best friend, Sarah, to go with her. "The thought of perhaps having to place my mother in a nursing home someday is nearly overwhelming to me," she says. "But I know I need to be realistic. I know that I will not be able to care for her at home if she reaches a state where she needs twenty-four-hour care. Sarah has been through this selection process before, for her father, and she knows the ropes and what to look for and what to ask. I feel so helpless! But one thing I know is that it's important to me for the nursing home to be close to my house so I can visit Mom every day. And of course it must provide good care."

When you have narrowed down your choices, it is time to meet with the administrator and, if possible, with other staff members so you can ask questions and voice any concerns. This is a time to have a written list of questions and, again, a friend or relative with you. Naturally, if the person with Alzheimer's is willing to attend this or any of your visits to nursing homes, please bring him or her along.

Here are some of the questions you may want to ask the administrator and other staff members when you have narrowed down your selection of a nursing home. There are literally hundreds of questions you can ask, and space does not permit us to list them all here. For sources of comprehensive lists of questions you can download and print out, see the section of appendix called "Finding and Evaluating Nursing Homes."

## Nursing Home Evaluation Checklist

### Staff

- What is the staff-to-resident ratio?

- Are resident requests (using the call bells) responded to in a timely manner (within 5 minutes)?

- Do the staff members treat residents with respect and courtesy? Are the residents spoken to as if they were children?

- Does the upper management (administrator, director of nursing, manager) appear to know the residents? Do they mingle with the residents often?

- Are there therapists and social workers on staff or does the facility contract out for these services?

- Does the staff appear to respect the privacy of residents (e.g., drawing the curtains while care is being administered, knocking before entering a room)?

- Does the facility have permanent full-time nurses and certified nurse assistants or does it use agency/registry staff?

### Resident Rooms

- How many residents share a room?

- Do the residents' rooms have windows?

- What amenities are in the rooms (e.g., bedside stand, reading light, comfortable chair, chest of drawers or adequate storage space)? Is the area for storing clothing and other items separate for each resident in a room?

- Can residents bring personal items from home, including furniture?

- Have residents personalized their rooms?

- Are call buttons easily accessible?

## Facility Environment

- Are there any obvious or overwhelming odors in the facility?

- Is the temperature comfortable? Do the residents' rooms have individual thermostats for heating and cooling?

- Is the facility clean, free of hazards, and well-lit?

- Is the furniture sturdy and comfortable?

- Are there handrails in the hallways?

- Does the facility have areas where residents and visitors can meet? Are these areas well maintained?

- Are there fire extinguishers visible? A sprinkler system?

- Are the bathrooms clean and conveniently located?

- How many residents share a bathroom?

- Are there rails or hand grips in the toilet and bathing areas?

- Is there a call button near the toilet?

- How often are residents bathed?

- Is the kitchen clean?

- Is the dining area clean, well-lit, and pleasant?

- Is the dining area large enough to accommodate most of the residents? Is there more than one dining area for residents? Are meals served in shifts?

## Meals (it is recommended that you visit during several meal times)

- Is there a weekly or monthly menu posted? How often are the options rotated?

- Is there a professional dietician on staff? Can you speak with him or her?

- Are residents offered alternatives to meet their dietary needs or preferences?

- Does the food look and smell appealing? Is it served at the proper temperature?

- Do the residents seem to enjoy the food?

- Are residents who need help with their meals being assisted in a timely fashion?

- What provisions are made for residents who are unable to go to the dining room?

## Appearance of Residents

- Are residents positioned comfortably in comfortable chairs? Are they provided trays or "lap buddies"?

- Are residents lined up in the hallways in wheelchairs and left alone for long periods of time?

- Are residents dressed for breakfast?

- Are residents well groomed (shaved, clean clothes, combed hair, trimmed nails)?

## Activities

- Is there a full-time activities director? Can you meet with this individual?

- Are activity calendars posted? Is there a broad range of activities?

- Are there activities for patients who are not able to leave their rooms?

- Are residents offered an opportunity to participate in religious services?

- How does the facility handle holidays and residents' birthdays?

- Does the facility bring in outside entertainment and activities?

Miscellaneous

- Does the facility regularly hold meetings that family members can attend and voice their opinions and ask questions?

- How often do physicians visit the facility?

- What hospital does the facility use in emergencies?

- What is the billing procedure? How accessible are the staff in the accounting department for questions and concerns?

- What are the results of the facility's last inspection by the Department of Public Health?

- How is personal laundry handled?

- What type of system is in place to handle wandering?

- Does the facility provide transportation to hospitals, doctor offices, or community functions? Is there an extra charge for this service?

## THE BOTTOM LINE

Over time, your loved one with Alzheimer's will need an increasing amount of care, and so now is the time to consider what living arrangement options you have at your disposal. Although planning ahead can be stressful for both you and the person with Alzheimer's, it can also bring you peace of mind, knowing that you are ensuring that your loved one will receive proper care and that he or she has an opportunity to participate in the decision-making process.

# CHAPTER 12

Get Outside Help

This chapter is dedicated to you, the caregivers—the daughters, sons, spouses, siblings, cousins, other relatives, and friends—who care for a person who has Alzheimer's disease. The challenges and emotional roller-coaster rides you experience every day can be overwhelming. True, some days are better than others. In fact, our hope is that because you are caring for someone who is in the early stages of the disease that you and your loved one are sharing many good days. We hope this book is helping with that goal.

But no matter how many good days there are, there is still the knowledge that the demands of caregiving will continue to increase as the disease progresses, and that you are always called upon, physically and emotionally, to meet those demands.

So are you taking care of yourself? Or are you so caught up in caring for your loved one that you forget to eat right, get enough sleep, relax, exercise, and generally be good to yourself?

In this chapter we discuss how you can get relief from the physical and emotional stress of caregiving.

# IT'S OKAY TO HAVE NEGATIVE FEELINGS

"I feel so guilty because I get angry and then yell at my mother," says Laura, who cares for her 71-year-old mother, Rebecca. "My brother will come over to visit us and he'll say, 'Well, she doesn't seem bad at all. Why do you get so upset?' And that drives me crazy. She doesn't live with him, she lives with me. And even though I know she can't help some of the things that she does, I have a hard time holding in my feelings. I don't want to take it out on her. I just don't think anyone understands what I'm going through."

It is very difficult for caregivers to accept that they will experience many negative feelings, such as frustration, anger, depression, and guilt, while they also love and care for the patient who has Alzheimer's disease. You are not a monster or a terrible person because you have these feelings; you are human, and these are normal reactions to a difficult situation.

Accepting the duality of negative feelings and your loving caregiving role is a daily balancing act. Once you do accept the challenge, you will be better able to deal with your negative feelings.

## Anger

Anger may be the most common emotion that caregivers experience. The sooner you accept that you are angry the sooner you will be able to manage it so that it does not manage you. "The last thing I wanted to do was direct my anger at my husband," says Irma. "So I found myself getting angry at the doctor, the pharmacist, the nurse, even the social worker. Like it was all their fault. Fortunately they understood, and the social worker was able to gently persuade me to talk to someone. She was really so patient with me, even while I was so impatient. So I started visiting my rabbi, and I'm feeling much better, less angry, and more accepting of the situation."

Anger is an emotion that is frequently misdirected, causing people to lash out at the person who has Alzheimer's disease, at other people (as Irma did), or at themselves. Some people repress their anger, directing it all inward. All of these scenarios place great stress on physical and emotional health and can lead to stomach disorders, headache, depression, fatigue, insomnia, and other problems. To avoid these and other negative responses to misdirected anger, you can try the following:

- Avoid or change situations that make you feel angry. For example, Bryan gets furious when his father goes into the garage and moves all of his tools around. "He misplaces them, loses them, he's even broken a thing or two," says Bryan. "I have lots of stuff hanging on the walls, in drawers and on shelves, so it's not all in one place. And if I lock Dad out of the garage, he gets anxious and I feel bad." Bryan's solution was to ask one of his father's friends to come over several times a week, and the two men are building cabinets for storing the tools. "It's a win-win," says Bryan. "Dad gets to handle the tools, which he loves to do, he and his friend are spending time together, and I'm getting a completely reorganized—and lockable—set of cabinets for my tools."

- If a feeling of anger becomes overwhelming, remove yourself from the situation, even if only briefly. Leave the room, go for a walk, listen to favorite music, call a friend, scream into a pillow—whatever it takes for you to relieve your anger in a safe way and in a way so that you are not lashing out physically or emotionally at the person with Alzheimer's, another person, or yourself.

- Exercise regularly, every day if possible. Physical activity is an excellent way to release pent-up tension and anger. Make exercise a priority.

- Seek outside help. You might contact someone in your support group, call a spiritual advisor, or go see a counselor or therapist. If you ever feel so angry that you are afraid you might physically harm the person who has Alzheimer's, get help immediately. Call an Alzheimer's Association representative or a professional counselor for help. Physical aggression against people with Alzheimer's disease is not uncommon among caregivers. You can get help.

## Embarrassment

Even during the early stages of Alzheimer's, the patient's behavior may occasionally be unpredictable or embarrassing. "My husband and I were in the supermarket," says Janice, "and when we got to the cereal section, Wes was suddenly overwhelmed by the number of choices of cereals. He began to panic and to say in an increasingly loud voice, 'I can't find it, I can't find it.' Everyone in the aisle was looking at us, and I was so embarrassed. I got panicky too, and I tried to find the cereal he wanted so I could make him stop. Fortunately I saw it and handed it to him, and he stopped yelling. I was humiliated and couldn't wait to leave the store."

If you are with family or friends and something embarrassing happens, you can explain that the behavior is out of the control of the patient. If something embarrassing happens when you are with strangers, it can be more difficult to accept. How to deal with embarrassing situations is a good topic to bring up in your support group or online support. You will quickly discover that you are not alone. Being a member of such a "club" may not solve your embarrassment problem, but it can certainly take the edge off.

## Guilt

It is easy for caregivers to let guilt get the upper hand and distort their ability to make rational decisions. Sally, for example, had decided that she was being selfish if she wanted some time for herself apart from caring for her mother at home, so she never accepted help from anyone. "Mom said she didn't want anyone else to come over to stay with her," says Sally. "She doesn't get upset when I go grocery shopping or I need to go out to get something for her, but she doesn't want me to go out any other time. She says she's afraid to be alone, and that the only person she wants to be around is me. I don't have a life."

Sally had convinced herself that if she insisted on going out for herself and found a suitable person to stay with her mother, that she would be guilty of neglecting her mother. It wasn't until one of her mother's friends, Barbara, came over one day and said that she would not leave until Sally went out for a while and did something for herself that Sally began to change her thinking. "When I got back from my two-hour respite," says Sally, "during which I felt so guilty and worried that my mother would be upset when I got home, I discovered my mother and Barbara having tea and laughing over some silly joke. My mother wasn't upset that I had gone out. Barbara said to me, 'See, you just have to put your foot down. You aren't asking for anything unfair. You need to get out.' So now

Barbara comes over once a week and I go out for the afternoon without feeling guilty!"

If you ever feel guilty, think about this:

• Did you yell at your loved one or someone else because you felt frustrated or scared or angry? Apologize and realize that you are human. Next time you feel angry, try one of the suggestions in the section "Anger."

• Did you go out and feel guilty when you got back? If you left the person with Alzheimer's in capable hands, then you have no reason to feel guilty. It is critical for you to have respite.

• Do you feel guilty because you get frustrated and angry with the person who has Alzheimer's and you have thoughts of wishing you could run away or not have the responsibility anymore? These are very common feelings. It can help to talk with others who are experiencing the same things— support group members. Utilize them, they can really save your sanity.

## SEEKING HELP FROM OTHERS

We hope you have accepted that as a caregiver, you cannot do it all, that no one else should expect you to, and that you should not even try. It is time to admit that when you feel you are about to be overwhelmed, you need to ask for help, that you need to take care of yourself, and that it is okay to ask for help. What are you going to do?

First, evaluate what your greatest needs are. Do you need help with housekeeping? Would you like someone to take over some or all of the responsibility for meals?

Do you need someone to stay with your loved one while you get away for a while? Would you like to share your feelings with others who know what it's like to be a caregiver? How about all of the above?

Rita was trying to do it all, and she had come to realize that it wasn't possible anymore. When her father first moved in with her, she worked out an arrangement with her job so she could work at home and just go into the office once a week. For that one day, Rita paid a neighbor to come in to stay with her father. But while Rita was at home, she found it very difficult to work. "Dad is still able to function rather well, but he is so needy. He follows me around the house or tries to talk to me while I'm working. It's reached the point where I'm saving my work until after he falls asleep, but then I'm so tired I can hardly keep my eyes open during the day. I'm so stressed that it's affecting my work, and I cannot afford to lose my job."

Geoff and his wife of 43 years, Felicia, still lived in the same house they bought when they first got married. When Felicia was diagnosed with early Alzheimer's nine months ago, Geoff, a 70-year-old retired production manager, was in great health, and he felt like he could easily handle Felicia and her needs.

"She was, and still is, able to do a lot for herself," says Geoff. "She can't prepare meals, but she doesn't need help eating. I take her shopping with me, and lately she's been more anxious when we're in the store, so I have to watch her carefully. We take walks just about every day when the weather is good, and she's more anxious about that, too. I guess her anxiety is just rubbing off on me, and I can't sleep very well anymore. I'm always worried about her. I want to be able to keep her here in this house as long as possible because it's full of memories and I think she feels safe here. I guess I feel safe here, too, but I'm just really tired."

Both Rita and Geoff are being overwhelmed by their caregiver responsibilities, and they need to reach out for help before they become ill and unable to care for their loved one or themselves. What are some of their—and your—options?

## Support Groups—Community and Cyberspace

"I don't know what I'd do without my Alzheimer's support group meetings," says Greta. "I go to two meetings each week, and the people are marvelous. They're so loving and understanding, and we all help each other. It's like a family. I feel uplifted when I leave there, even though we are all dealing with such a terrible disease. But at least we can share with each other, and it means so much."

Alzheimer's support groups are very popular and can be found in nearly every city in the United States. Your local Alzheimer's Association chapter will be able to tell you where to find the groups in your area, the times they meet, and how to contact them. If you want to add another level of support, then you might also think about joining an online support group.

In recent years, there has been an explosion of Internet chats, blogs, and online support groups where caregivers can reach out and "touch" someone through the magic of cyberspace communication. We still believe face-to-face interaction is much better than the virtual approach, but getting support on the Internet has its advantages.

One is time: You can get online any time of the day or night and likely find someone in an online support group who will either chat with you, or you can type your messages and then wait for a response later. You can also send and receive e-mails at any hour, or you can start a blog or respond to others' blogs.

Online support groups and chats are good "fill-ins" for when you can't get out of the house. They are also an alternative when you want to talk to someone but there's no one else available at the moment in your "real" life.

Naturally, you should be careful of the groups and chats that you join. Once again, the Alzheimer's Association is a great place to begin, as the organization has an active online support system. You can also ask friends, relatives, and best of all, other support group members about any online groups that they frequent. See the appendix for online support group addresses you can try. Many of these online support groups also provide lots of information on Alzheimer's research, legal matters, long-distance caregiving, how to cope with behavioral issues, and much more.

## Counseling

Some day you may decide you want to talk with a professional about your feelings of frustration, anger, or depression. Perhaps you would feel safer or more comfortable sharing your feelings with someone who has been trained in helping caregivers sort through the overwhelming emotions that come with the job. Counselors, therapists (marriage, family, or general), psychologists, psychiatrists, and clergy are all possibilities.

You may have the option of either individual or group sessions. A group session allows you to explore your feelings under professional guidance while sharing them with others who are in a situation similar to yours. In one way such sessions are like a support group, but here you have the advantage of getting professional guidance.

If you need help finding a professional, ask your social worker, doctor, nurse, or a representative of the Alzheimer's Association for the names of people who work with caregivers and family members of Alzheimer's patients. Your local Area Agencies on Aging may also have some suggestions.

## Family, Friends, and Others

Alzheimer's disease can be an isolating condition. It is not unusual for caregivers and family members to notice a decline in the number of friends, neighbors, and other family members as well who stop calling or coming over once they learn about a diagnosis of Alzheimer's disease. When these people stay away from you and your loved one, you may feel isolated and like people don't care. But often people stay away because they don't know what to say or they don't realize that you are having a difficult time. You may have to take the first step and let them know that you miss their company and their phone calls.

You know what they say about a squeaky wheel, so let people know that you could use some help. Don't feel guilty about burdening them. If you let family and good friends know that you need some respite, you may get more response than you expect. If several people offer to assist you, set up a schedule.

Some church and volunteer groups provide volunteers who visit with people who are home-bound. Oscar found one such group at his wife's church. "There's a group of older men and women at Milly's church who will send someone over to the house to stay with her while I go out for a few hours," says Oscar. "I have a chance to spend one afternoon a week doing whatever I want to do. I felt a little guilty at first, but Milly and Priscilla, the woman who's been coming over, play cards and talk or make jig-saw puzzles together, and she seems to be having a good time."

## Caring for the Caregiver

Finally, we want to leave you with a prescription for caring for the caregiver. Studies show that caregiver stress takes a significant toll on the spouses, daughters, sons, and other caregivers, often eventually resulting in illness. In a recent study published in *Health and Quality of Life Outcomes,* an evaluation of caregivers showed that 53 percent had little time for themselves, 55 percent observed their own worsening health, 56 percent were tired, and 51 percent were not getting enough sleep. Please do not let this happen to you.

- **Nourish your body**. Poor diet, along with chronic stress, can take a huge toll on your immune system and quickly cause illness. You want your loved one to eat well, so you should too. Keep easy and nutritious foods in the house so you won't feel the pressure of having to prepare something if you are too tired. Fresh fruits such as grapes, berries, and bananas are easy to eat. Keep dried fruits, dry roasted nuts, 100% vegetable juices, yogurt, whole-grain crackers, and snackable vegetables such as baby carrots, celery, cherry tomatoes, bell peppers, and cucumbers on hand. Many restaurants and supermarkets will deliver meals for a nominal fee.

- **Schedule respite time**. Have at least one significant block of time each week—three or four hours or more—when you can get away from the caregiving environment and do what you want to do. This is a time when you can call upon friends, family, or a volunteer group to help. This respite time can also mean that the person with Alzheimer's goes on an outing while you stay at home. Allie is grateful for her "free Sundays," as she calls them. "Each Sunday, either our son or daughter comes over and takes their father out for most of the day. I stay home or I go out—whatever

I want to do, it's my time. I so look forward to Sundays!"

- **Continue with your hobbies and interests**. If you enjoy gardening, don't stop. If you like going to book reading groups, make arrangements so you can continue to do so. You may need to make some compromises on some activities, but you should not stop doing things that make you feel fulfilled.

- **Practice stress reduction every day**. There are many things you can do at home to reduce the level of stress in your life. Take 15 to 20 minutes to meditate or do deep breathing exercises, yoga, or visualization. You might share this with the person who has Alzheimer's, as it can reduce his or her level of uncertainty and anxiety as well.

- **Socialize**. Do not isolate yourself from others. Find a class, support group, church group, health club, or any place where you can talk and mingle with others. Invite neighbors or friends over for coffee.

- **Consider volunteer work**. This is not only a great way to socialize, but it can also make you feel fulfilled. Do you love animals? Perhaps you can volunteer to walk dogs at the shelter a few hours each week. Do you love children? Maybe you could help at a local children's hospital ward or read to kids at the library.

- **Keep a journal or diary**. Many people find that writing down how they feel is cathartic and gives them perspective.

- **Take care of your spiritual side**. You might connect with a church, spiritual group, synagogue, temple, or meditation center—whatever path helps you feel more at peace and content.

- **Exercise**. Regular physical activity relieves stress as well as helps maintain physical conditioning. Take time to walk, jog, do yoga, or go to a gym. If it is difficult for you to get out of the house, invest in a treadmill, exercise bike, or other equipment. Used equipment can often be purchased for reasonable prices.

## THE BOTTOM LINE

It's simple: If you don't take care of the caregiver, who will? It is critically important that you maintain your physical, emotional, and spiritual well-being both for yourself and for the person who has Alzheimer's disease. Don't be afraid to reach out. Someone will be there to take your hand: a friend, relative, support group member, minister, fellow volunteer, a chat room cyberfriend. You are not alone.

# CHAPTER NOTES

## Chapter 1

Wang DO et al. Synapse- and stimulus-specific local translation during long-term neuronal plasticity. *Science* 2009 Jun 19; 324(5934): 1536–40.

Dolcos F et al. Remembering one year later: role of the amygdala and the medial temporal lobe memory system in retrieving emotional memories. *Proc Natl Acad Sci USA* 2005 Feb 15; 102(7): 2626–31.

## Chapter 2

Maki PM, Sundermann E. Hormone therapy and cognitive function. *Hum Reprod Update* 2009 May 25.

Mukamal KJ et al. Prospective study of alcohol consumption and risk of dementia in older adults. *JAMA* 2003 Mar 19; 289(11): 11405–13.

Oh, RC, Brown DL. Vitamin B$_{12}$ deficiency. *Am Fam Physician* 2003; 67:979–86.

Prakash A, Kumar A. Effect of N-acetyl cysteine against aluminum-induced cognitive dysfunction and oxidative damage in rats. *Basic Clin Pharmacol Toxicol* 2009 Mar 27.

Rondeau V et al. Aluminum and silica in drinking water and the risk of Alzheimer's disease or cognitive decline: findings from 15-year follow-up of the PAQUID cohort. *Am J Epidemiol* 2009 Feb 15; 169(4): 489–96.

Yaffe et al. Post-traumatic stress disorder and risk of dementia among US veterans. *Alzheimers Dementia* 2009; 5(4).

## Chapter 3

Burns DH et al. Near-infrared spectroscopy of blood plasma for diagnosis of sporadic Alzheimer disease. *J Alzheimers Dis* 2009 Jun 8; 17(2).

Cogswell JP et al. Identification of miRNA changes in Alzheimer's disease brain and CSF yields putative biomarkers and insights into disease pathways. *J Alzheimers Dis* 2008 May; 14(1): 27–41.

Hakansson K et al. Association between mid-life marital status and cognitive function in later life: population based cohort study. *BMJ* 2009 Jul 2; 339.

Kovacevic S et al. High-throughput, fully automated volumetry for prediction of MMSE and CDR decline in mild cognitive impairment. *Alzheimer Dis Assoc Disord* 2009 Apr-Jun; 23(2): 139–45.

# Chapter 4

Buchman AS et al. Total daily activity is associated with cognition in older persons. *Am J Geriatr Psychiatry* 2008 Aug; 16(8): 697–701.

Burns JM et al. Cardiorespiratory fitness and brain atrophy in early Alzheimer disease. *Neurology* 2008 Jul 15; 71(3): 210–16.

Deeny SP et al. Exercise, APOE, and working memory: MEG and behavioral evidence for benefit of exercise in epsilon4 carriers. *Biol Psychol* 2008; 78:179–87.

Etnier JL et al. Cognitive performance in older women relative to APoE-epsilon4 genotype and aerobic fitness. *Med Sci Sports Exerc* 2007; 39:199–207.

Green KN et al. Glucocorticoids increase amyloid-beta and tau pathology in a mouse model of Alzheimer's disease. *J Neurosci* 2006 Aug 30; 26(35): 9047–56.

Jackson et al. Dementia literacy: Public understanding of known risk factors. *Alzheimers Dementia* 2009; 5(4):410.

Loerbroks A et al. Nocturnal sleep duration and cognitive impairment in a population-based study of older adults. *Int J Geriatr Psychiatry* 2009 Jun 22.

Morch LS et al. Hormone therapy and ovarian cancer. *JAMA* 2009 Jul 15; 302(3): 298–305.

Perez CA et al. Benefits of physical exercise for older adults with Alzheimer's disease. *Geriatr Nurs* 2008 Nov–Dec; 29(6): 384–91.

Quinn et al. A clinical trial of docosahexanoic acid (DHA) for the treatment of Alzheimer's disease. *Alzheimers and Dementia* 2009 Jul; 5(4): 84.

Schuit AJ et al. Physical activity and cognitive decline, the role of the apolipoprotein e4 allele. *Med Sci Sports Exerc* 2001; 33:772–77.

Sing KM et al. Angiotensin-converting enzyme inhibitors and cognitive decline in older adults with hypertension: results from the cardiovascular health study. *Arch Intern Med* 2009 Jul 13; 169(13): 1195–202.

Steinberg M et al. Evaluation of a home-based exercise program in the treatment of Alzheimer's disease: the Maximizing Independence in Dementia (MIND) study. *Int J Geriatr Psychiatry* 2009 Jul; 24(7): 680–85.

Sterpenich V et al. Sleep promotes the neural reorganization of remote emotional memory. *J Neurosci* 2009 Apr 22; 29(16): 5143–52.

Wengreen et al. DASH diet adherence scores and cognitive decline and dementia among aging men and women: Cache County study of memory health and aging. *Alzheimers and Dementia* 2009 Jul; 5(4):128.

Van Praag H. Exercise and the brain: something to chew on. *Trends Neurosci* 2009 May; 32(5): 283–90.

Yurko-Mauro et al. Results of the MIDAS trial: Effects of docosahexaenoic acid on physiological and safety parameters in age-related cognitive decline. *Alzheimers and Dementia* 2009 Jul; 5(4): 84.

# Chapter 5

Breitner JC et al. Risk of dementia and AD with prior exposure to NSAIDs in an elderly community-based cohort. *Neurology* 2009 Jun 2; 72(22): 1899–905.

Doody RS et al. Effect of dimebon on cognition, activities of daily living, behavior, and global function in patients with mild-to-moderate Alzheimer's disease: a randomized, double-blind, placebo-controlled study. *Lancet* 2008 July 19; 372(9634): 207–15.

Duron E et al. Effects of antihypertensive therapy on cognitive decline in Alzheimer's disease. *Am J Hypertens* 2009 Jul 9.

Ebadi M et al. Therapeutic efficacy of selegiline in neurodegenerative disorders and neurological diseases. *Curr Drug Targets* 2006 Nov; 7(11): 1513–29.

Gauthier S. Dimebon improves cognitive function in people with mild to moderate Alzheimer's disease. *Evid Based Ment Health* 2009 Feb; 12(1); 21.

Gauthier S et al. Effect of tramiprostate in patients with mild-to-moderate Alzheimer's disease: exploratory analyses of the MIR sub-group of the Alphase Study. *J Nutr Health Aging* 2009 Jul; 13(6): 550–57.

Imbimbo BP. An update on the efficacy of non-steroidal anti-inflammatory drugs in Alzheimer's disease. *Expert Opin Investig Drugs* 2009 Aug; 18(8): 1147–68.

Kandiah N, Feldman HH. Therapeutic potential of statins in Alzheimer's disease. *J Neurol Sci* 2009 Aug 15; 283-(1–2): 230–34.

Li G et al. Statin therapy is associated with reduced neuropathologic changes in Alzheimer's disease. *Neurology* 2007 (69):878–85.

Lu PH et al. Donepezil delays progression to AD in MCI subjects with depressive symptoms. *Neurology* 2009 Jun 16; 72(24): 2115–21.

Pasqualetti P et al. A randomized controlled study on effects of ibuprofen on cognitive progression of Alzheimer's disease. *Aging Clin Exp Res* 2009 Apr; 21(2): 102–10.

Tsunekawa H et al. Synergistic effects of selegiline and donepezil on cognitive impairment induced by amyloid beta (25–35). *Behav Brain Res* 2008 Jul 19; 190(2): 224–32.

## Chapter 6

Cole GM et al. Omega-3 fatty acids and dementia. *Prostaglandins Leukot Essent Fatty Acids* 2009 Jun 10.

Desilets AR et al. Role of huperzine A in the treatment of Alzheimer's disease. *Ann Pharmacother* 2009 Mar; 43(3): 514–18.

Fotuhi M et al. Fish consumption, long-chair omega-3 fatty acids and risk of cognitive decline or Alzheimer disease: a complex association. *Nat Clin Pract Neurol* 2009 Mar; 5(3): 140–52.

Frautschy SA et al. Phenolic anti-inflammatory antioxidant reversal of Abeta-induced cognitive deficits and neuropathology. *Neurobiol Aging* 2001; 22(6): 993–1005.

Ishrat T et al. Amelioration of cognitive deficits and neurodegeneration by curcumin in rat model of sporadic dementia of Alzehimer's type (SDAT). *Eur Neuropsychopharmacol* 2009 Mar 27.

Kasper S, Schubert H. Ginkgo biloba extract EGb 761R in the treatment of dementia: evidence of efficacy and tolerability. *Fortschr Neurol Psychiatr* 2009 Jul 20.

Kronenberg G et al. Folic acid, neurodegenerative and neuropsychiatric disease. *Curr Mol Med* 2009 Apr; 9(3): 315–23.

Li J et al. Huperzine A for Alzheimer's disease. *Cochrane Database Syst Rev* 2008 Apr 16; (2): CD005592.

Lim GP et al. The curry spice curcumin reduces oxidative damage and amyloid pathology in an Alzheimer transgenic mouse. *J Neurosci* 2001 Nov 1; 21(21): 8370–77.

Lloret A et al. Vitamin E paradox in Alzheimer's disease: it does not prevent loss of cognition and may even be detrimental. *J Alzheimers Dis* 2009 May; 17(1): 143–49.

Pan R et al. Curcumin improves learning and memory ability and its neuroprotective mechanism in mice. *Chin Med J* 2008 121(9): 832–39.

Tchantchou F, Shea TB. Folate deprivation, the methionine cycle, and Alzheimer's disease. *Vitam Horm* 2008; 79:83–97.

Xu SS et al. Efficacy of tablet huperzine-A on memory, cognition and behavior in Alzheimer's disease. *Chung Kuo Yao Li Hsueh Pao* 1995 Sep; 16 (5):391–95.

Yang F et al. Curcumin inhibits formation of amyloid beta oligomers and fibrils, binds plaques, and reduces amyloid in vivo. *J Biol Chem* 2005 Feb 18; 280(7): 5892–5901.

## Chapter 8

Aveyard B, et al. Therapeutic touch in dementia care. *Nurs Older People.* 2002; 14(6):20–21.

Diaz, J. Breath, Lives, Memory. *Boston Globe* Sept. 30, 2008.

Janata P. The neural architecture of music-evoked autobiographical memories. *Cerebral Cortex* 2009 Feb 24.

Verghese J. Cognitive and mobility profile of older social dancers. *J Am Geriatr Soc* 2006 Aug; 54(8): 1241–44.

Woods DL, et al. The effect of therapeutic touch on behavioral symptoms of persons with dementia. *Altern Ther Health Med* 2005; 11(1): 66–74.

Woods, DL and M. Dimond. The effect of therapeutic touch on agitated behavior and cortisol in persons with Alzheimer's disease. *Biol Res Nurs* 2002; 4(2): 104–14.

## Chapter 9

Weil, Andrew. "Learning a Foreign Language Can Help You Live Longer," *ABC News*, October 23, 2005.

## Chapter 12

Dang S et al. The dementia caregiver—a primary care approach. *South Med J* 2008 Dec; 101(12): 1246–51.

Ferrara M et al. Prevalence of stress, anxiety, and depression in with Alzheimer caregivers. *Health Qual Life Outcomes* 2008 Nov 6; 6:93.

Losada A et al. Leisure and distress in caregivers for elderly patients. *Arch Gerontol Geriatr* 2009 Jun 30.

Scholzel-Dorenbos CJ et al. Quality of life and burden of spouses of Alzheimer disease patients. *Alzheimer Dis Assoc Disord* 2009 Apr–Jun; 23(2): 171–77.

Skinner K. Nursing interventions to assist in decreasing stress in caregivers of Alzheimer's patients. *ABNF J* 2009 Winter; 20(1): 22–24.

# APPENDIX

Information About Alzheimer's Disease and Caregiving


## Alzheimer's Association

www.alz.org/index.asp

The leading voluntary health organization dedicated to care, support and research of Alzheimer's disease.

## Alzheimer's Disease Education and Referral Center (ADEAR)

www.nia.nih.gov/alzheimers

Offers the latest information and research on Alzheimer's disease.

## Alzheimer's Foundation of America

www.alzfdn.org

The Foundation's mission is to provide care and services

to people confronting dementia through member organizations dedicated to improving quality of life.

## Alzheimer's Research and Prevention Foundation

www.alzheimersprevention.org

An organization dedicated to reducing the incidence of Alzheimer's disease by conducting clinical research and providing educational outreach.

## The Brain Matters

www.thebrainmatters.org

This is the American Academy of Neurology's public website, providing the latest information and resources on specific neurologic disorders.

## National Alliance for Caregiving

www.caregiving.org

A nonprofit that provides videos, websites, fact sheets, and other resources addressing the issues faced by family caregivers.

## National Family Caregivers Association

www.nfcacares.org

A grassroots organization that provides family caregivers with support, information, and practical resources.

# ALZHEIMER'S DISEASE SUPPORT GROUPS: ONLINE

## Alzheimer's Association Online Community

alzheimers.infopop.cc/eve

Provides several forums for caregivers, people with memory loss, and health professionals. Users can ask questions of care consultants.

## Alzheimer's Caregiver Support Online

alzonline.phhp.ufl.edu

An Internet- and telephone-based support network for caregivers of people with dementia. Offers online caregiver education and support classes and links to Alzheimer's caregiver resources in your local area.

## Care-givers.com

www.care-givers.com

Online support for caregivers.

## Empowering Caregivers

www.care-givers.com/pages/resources/online/
care-sites.html

Offers many resources from message boards to chat, journal-writing exercises, and information on alternative healing.

# Healingwell

www.healingwell.com/alzheimers

A website that offers interactive tools for caregivers and patients. Features message boards and chat rooms, newsletters, and resource directories.

# TheAlzheimerSpouse.com

www.thealzheimerspouse.com

This website focuses on helping the spouses of Alzheimer's patients and features blogs, message boards, booklists, and information on how to cope with the impact of Alzheimer's on marriage and partnership.

# FINDING AND EVALUATING NURSING HOMES

The Health and Human Services Medicare website (www.medicare.gov/Nursing/Overview.asp) offers information on nursing homes, including how to compare them, about nursing home inspections, how to pay for care, and other important details.

The Alzheimer's Association provides a checklist for evaluating nursing homes and a database of nursing homes, as well as much more information at
www.alzinfo.org/providers/default.aspx?AreaId=3
and
www.alzinfo.org/pdfs/checklist.pdf.

The Aging Parents and Elder Care website offers a

comprehensive checklist for selecting a nursing home/
skilled nursing facility:

www.aging-parents-and-elder-care.com/Pages/Checklists/
Nursing_Home_Checklist.html

## LEGAL ADVICE

An Alzheimer's Association office can suggest elder law
attorneys in your area. Call 800-272-3900 to find your
local office.

Free legal advice may be available in your area. Contact
your local Area Agency on Aging or the Eldercare Loca-
tor at 800-677-1116 or www.eldercare.gov.

### National Academy of Elder Law Attorneys

www.naela.org

Provides access to a list of elder law attorneys in the United
States

## BRAIN GAMES
Online sources of brain games.

### Brain.com

www.brain.com/brain_games2.htm

### Brainist.com

brainist.com/

## Everyday Health

www.everydayhealth.com

## Games for the Brain

www.gamesforthebrain.com/

## Lumosity: Reclaim Your Brain

www.lumosity.com/

## The Original Memory Gym

www.memorise.org/

## Prevention.com

www.prevention.com/cda/categorypage.do?channel=
health&category=brain.fitness&topic=brain.games

# GLOSSARY

**Allele:** A form of a gene. Every person receives two alleles of a gene, one from each parent. The apolipoprotein E (APOE) gene has three common alleles: E2, E3, and E4.

**Apolipoprotein E (APOE) gene:** A gene located on chromosome 19 that is involved in the production of a protein that helps carry cholesterol in the bloodstream. The APOE4 allele is considered a risk factor for Alzheimer's disease.

**Beta-amyloid:** A type of protein that accumulates in the brain and forms deposits that contribute to the destruction of brain cells (neurons).

**Biomarker:** A substance or characteristic that can be measured objectively and is an indicator of normal body processes, disease processes, or the body response to therapy. For example, blood pressure is a biomarker that indicates risk of heart disease.

**Cerebral cortex:** The part of the brain involved with

language, learning, reasoning, and other high-functioning processes.

**Cholinesterase inhibitors:** Medications that help preserve the brain levels of the neurotransmitter acetylcholine and thus help maintain cognitive functioning.

**Chromosome:** A structure that contains DNA and proteins and is found in nearly all the cells of the body. Chromosomes carry genes, which direct the cell to make proteins.

**Cognitive function:** High-level brain activities, such as reasoning, remembering, speaking, reading, decision-making, writing, and abstract thinking.

**Cortisol:** A hormone made and secreted by the adrenal glands in response to physical or psychological stress.

**Dementia:** A general term used to describe any irreversible condition in which there is a decline in mental abilities caused by the death of nerve cells.

**Dopamine:** A neurotransmitter in the brain that causes brain dysfunction and disease when its levels are out of balance.

**Estrogen:** A naturally occurring hormone that may reduce the risk of developing Alzheimer's disease when given to postmenopausal women.

**Folic acid:** A B vitamin that appears to have a role in helping to prevent Alzheimer's disease.

**Frontal lobe:** An area in the front of the brain that is involved in controlling the ability to coordinate thoughts, planning, and scheduling.

**Galantamine:** One of the cholinesterase inhibitors used to treat Alzheimer's disease.

**Ginkgo biloba:** A Chinese herb that may help in the treatment of memory loss.

**Glutamate:** A neurotransmitter that is involved in memory and learning.

**Hippocampus:** An area of the brain, located deep in the temporal lobe, that is involved in learning and memory.

**Melatonin:** A hormone that is secreted by the pineal gland and is involved in the regulation of the sleep-wake cycle.

**Memantine:** A drug that has an impact on certain receptors in the brain (N-methyl-D-aspartate) and is helpful in treating Alzheimer's disease.

**Mild cognitive impairment:** A condition that causes slight problems with memory and other cognitive functions, but it is not serious enough to reduce an individual's ability to live independently.

**Neuron:** A nerve or brain cell.

**Neurotransmitter:** A chemical in the brain that helps neurons communicate with each other.

**Oxidative stress:** The damage inflicted upon the cells by free radicals when oxygen interacts with other substances in the body.

**Parietal lobe:** The area of the brain that is located behind and above the temporal lobe.

**Rivastigmine:** One of the cholinesterase inhibitors used to treat Alzheimer's disease.

**Selegiline:** A drug that has antioxidant properties and can be helpful in delaying the functional decline associated with Alzheimer's disease.

**Serotonin:** A neurotransmitter found in abnormally low levels in people who have Alzheimer's disease and depression.

**Statins:** Drugs designed to lower high cholesterol levels.

**Tangles:** The accumulation of abnormal hair-like protein clumps in nerve cells in the brain.

**Tau protein:** The main protein that makes up the tangles found in the brains of people who have Alzheimer's disease.